International Archives of Allergy and Immunology

Official Journal of the

Collegium Internationale Allergologicum

COLLEGIUM INTERNATIONALE CIA ALLERGOLOGICUM

Founded 1950 by D. Harley, P. Kallós, W. Löffler and F.W. Wittich
Continued by E.A. Brown (1952–1954), W. Kaufman (1955–1967), F. Hahn (1961–1972), H.C. Goodman (1963–1975), R.R.A. Coombs (1955–1984), Z. Trnka (1972–1987), P. Kallós (1950–1988), G.B. West (1959–1991), J. Bienenstock (1990–1991), L.Å. Hanson (1981–1991), K. Kano (1982–1991), F. Milgrom (1965–1991), K. Rother (1982–1991), G. Wick (1991–1997), B. Grubeck-Loebenstein (1991–1997), D. Kraft (1998–2002)

KARGER

Printed in Switzerland on acid-free and non-aging paper (ISO 9706) by Reinhardt Druck, Basel

Appears monthly: 3 volumes per year (12 issues)

Guidelines for Authors

International Archives of
Allergy and Immunology

'International Archives of Allergy and Immunology' appears monthly and provides a forum for publication of work from all aspects of modern allergology and immunology. Papers considered of special interest will be treated as 'hot topics' and every attempt will be made to publish these especially fast. The Editor-in-Chief, the Managing Editor and a team of internationally established Associate Editors competently covering all fields of allergology and immunology are responsible for the scientific quality of this international core journal. *International Archives* publishes original work in the fields of allergy, immunopathology and transplantation, cellular immunology, immunogenetics, immunopharmacology and immunoendocrinology, mucosal immunity, immunology of infectious diseases and immunology of connective tissue diseases. In addition, reviews, minireviews, commentaries and opinions on controversial subjects are published regularly. A new system of manuscript submission, reviewing and processing guarantees competent and fair reviewing as well as fast and high quality publication.

Submission

Only papers written in English are considered. Manuscript submissions to the 'International Archives of Allergy and Immunology' are now online! Detailed Online Submission Instructions with a link to the Submission Website are at http://www.karger.com/iaa/. Before submitting your manuscript, you are encouraged to review the detailed guidelines at www.karger.com/iaa_guidelines for specific directions as how to get a manuscript ready for submission. If you should have any problems with your submission, or should you feel the need to submit the paper in a non-electronic form, please contact the editorial office:

Prof. Dr. R. Valenta
Editor-in-Chief
S. Karger AG
Editorial Office 'International Archives of Allergy and Immunology'
PO Box
CH–4009 Basel (Switzerland)
Tel. +41 61 306 1360
Fax +41 61 306 1434
E-Mail e.lieberherr@karger.ch

Mailing address for courier deliveries only:
Allschwilerstr. 10
CH–4055 Basel (Switzerland)

Original papers: Submitted manuscripts should be fully documented reports of original research. They must describe significant and original observations to be critically evaluated and, if necessary, repeated.

Short communications: These manuscripts should not contain more than ***2 printed pages (i.e. 6,460 characters per page)***, including an abstract, essential references and not more than 3 tables or figures. Such communications should represent complete, original studies and should be arranged in the same way as full-length manuscripts.

Novel Insights from Clinical Practice (formerly Case Reports): The publication space available for case reports is very limited. The journal only considers case reports with significant new insights or with an extremely unusual and memorable course. Highlighted boxes containing one or two bullet points on 'Established facts' (what is already known) and 'Novel insights' (what new information has been gained) are required and should be placed on the first page of the report. These should be selected so as to reinforce the novelty of the clinical observation. The manuscript should be presented with an abstract (unstructured, max. 200 words), followed by introduction, case report and discussion. Maximum 3 figures.

Review articles, minireviews, opinion articles, controversies and commentaries: Authors who wish to contribute a manuscript to one of these categories should contact the Editor-in-Chief. Minireviews should be focused, brief reports on topics of current interest. Commentaries should offer a more personalized perspective on a topic that will be of interest to the general readership. All contributions to these categories will be subject to Editorial review.

Letters to the Editor concerning work published in the journal may be submitted. They should not exceed 2 manuscript pages including one table or figure.

Conditions

All manuscripts are subject to editorial review. Manuscripts are received with the explicit understanding that they are not under simultaneous consideration by any other publication. A cover letter with the name, address, and telephone and telefax numbers of the corresponding author must accompany each manuscript. This letter must include a statement that affirms that all authors agree with the submission. Submission of an article for publication implies the transfer of the copyright from the author to the publisher upon acceptance. Accepted papers become the permanent property of *International Archives of Allergy and Immunology* and may not be reproduced by any means, in whole or in part, without the written consent of the publisher. It is the author's responsibility to obtain permission to reproduce illustrations, tables, etc. from other publications. One of the criteria considered in reviewing manuscripts is the proper treatment of animals. In particular, the use of painful or otherwise noxious stimuli must be carefully and thoroughly justified. Papers that do not meet these criteria will not be accepted for publication.

Arrangement

Manuscripts should be written in English and be as concise as possible.
Be sure to display line numbers (1, 2, 3, and so forth) in the left margin of the manuscript (line numbering can be added from the Page Setup or Format menu of word processing programs). The line numbering should be continuous throughout the entire manuscript, from the title page through to the final page (i.e., do not begin numbering from 1 again at the top of each page).

Title page: The first page of each paper should indicate the title, the authors' full names, affiliations and e-mail addresses, the institute where the work was conducted, and a short title for use as running head. NB: Authors wishing to preserve the phonetic meaning of diacritics (PubMed reduces diacritics to their root characters) must spell their names accordingly when submitting manuscripts (e.g. Müller should be Mueller).

Full address: The exact postal address of the corresponding author complete with postal code must be given at the bottom of the title page. Please also supply phone and fax numbers, as well as an e-mail address.

Key words: A list of 3–10 key words should be included for indexing purposes.

Abstract: **Provide on a separate page an abstract of not more than 250 words. This abstract should consist of four paragraphs, labeled Background, Methods, Results, and Conclusions. They should briefly describe, respectively, the problem being addressed in the study, how the study was performed, the salient results, and what the authors conclude from the results.**

The text should be arranged in the following sections: Introduction, Material and Methods, Results, Discussion, Acknowledgement, References.

Footnotes: Avoid footnotes. When essential, they are numbered consecutively and typed at the foot of the appropriate page.

Tables and illustrations: Tables and illustrations (both numbered in Arabic numerals) should be prepared on separate pages. Tables require a heading and figures a legend, also prepared on a separate page. For the reproduction of illustrations, only good drawings and original photographs can be accepted; negatives or photocopies cannot be used. Due to technical reasons, figures with a screen background should not be submitted. When possible, group several illustrations on one block for reproduction (max. size 180 × 223 mm) or provide crop marks. Each illustration must be labeled with its number and the author's name. Electronically submitted b/w half-tone and color illustrations must have a final resolution of 300 dpi after scaling (final size), line drawings one of 800–1,200 dpi. Figure files must not be embedded in a document file but submitted separately (see detailed instructions at www.karger.com/iaa/).

Color illustrations
Online edition: Color illustrations are reproduced free of charge. In the print version, the illustrations are reproduced in black and white. Please avoid referring to the colors in the text and figure legends.
Print edition: Up to 6 color illustrations per page can be integrated within the text at CHF 800.– per page.

Abbreviations: Avoid overuse of abbreviations. Introduce an abbreviation only when the same term occurs three or more times.

KARGER

Fax +41 61 306 12 34
E-Mail karger@karger.ch
www.karger.com

The Guidelines for Authors are available at:
www.karger.com/iaa_Guidelines

References: In the text identify references by Arabic numerals [in square brackets]. Material submitted for publication but not yet accepted should be noted as 'unpublished data' and not be included in the reference list. The list of references should include only those publications which are cited in the text. Do not alphabetize; number references in the order in which they are first mentioned in the text. The surnames of the authors followed by initials should be given. There should be no punctuation other than a comma to separate the authors. Preferably, please cite all authors. Abbreviate journal names according to the Index Medicus system. (Also see International Committee of Medical Journal Editors: Uniform requirements for manuscripts submitted to biomedical journals. N Engl J Med 1997;336:309–315 or www.icmje.org).

Examples

(a) Papers published in periodicals: Sun J, Koto H, Chung KF: Interaction of ozone and allergen challenges on bronchial responsiveness and inflammation in sensitised guinea pigs. Int Arch Allergy Immunol 1997;112:191–195.

(b) Papers published only with DOI numbers: Theoharides TC, Boucher W, Spear K: Serum interleukin-6 reflects disease severity and osteoporosis in mastocytosis patients. Int Arch Allergy Immunol DOI: 10.1159/000063858.

(c) Monographs: Matthews DE, Farewell VT: Using and Understanding Medical Statistics, ed 3, revised. Basel, Karger, 1996.

(d) Edited books: Parren PWHI, Burton DR: Antibodies against HIV-1 from phage display libraries: Mapping of an immune response and progress towards antiviral immunotherapy; in Capra JD (ed): Antibody Engineering. Chem Immunol. Basel, Karger, 1997, vol 65, pp 18–56.

Full address: The exact postal address complete with postal code must be given at the bottom of the title page. Please also supply phone and fax numbers, as well as your e-mail address.

Reference Management Software: Use of EndNote is recommended for easy management and formatting of citations and reference lists.

Digital Object Identifier (DOI)

S. Karger Publishers supports DOIs as unique identifiers for articles. A DOI number will be printed on the title page of each article. DOIs can be useful in the future for identifying and citing articles published online without volume or issue information. More information can be found at www.doi.org.

Author's Choice™

Karger's Author's Choice service broadens the reach of your article and gives all users worldwide free and full access for reading, downloading and printing at www.Karger.com. The option is available for a one-time fee of CHF 3000.–, which is a permissible cost in grant allocation. More information can be found at www.karger.com/authors_choice.

NIH-Funded Research

The U.S. National Institutes of Health (NIH) mandates under the NIH Public Access Policy that final, peer-reviewed manuscripts appear in its digital database within 12 months of the official publication date. As a service to authors, Karger submits the final version of your article on your behalf to PubMed Central. For those selecting our premium Author's Choice service, we will send your article immediately upon publishing, accelerating the accessibility of your work without the usual embargo. More details on NIH's Public Access Policy is available at http://publicaccess.nih.gov/FAQ.htm#a1

Self-Archiving

Karger permits authors to archive their pre-prints (i.e. pre-refereeing) or post-prints (i.e. final draft post-refereeing) on their personal or institution's servers, provided the following conditions are met: Articles may not be used for commercial purposes, must be linked to the publisher's version, and must acknowledge the publisher's copyright. Authors selecting Karger's Author's Choice feature, however, are also permitted to archive the final, published version of their article, which includes copyediting and design improvements as well as citation links.

Page Charges

There are no page charges for papers of 5 or fewer printed pages (including tables, illustrations and references). Each additional complete or partial page is charged to the author at CHF 325.–. The allotted size of a paper is 5 printed pages (6,460 characters per page), which is equal to approx. 14 manuscript pages including tables, illustrations and references.

Proofs

Unless indicated otherwise, proofs are sent to the first-named author and should be returned with the least possible delay. Alterations made in proofs, other than the correction of printer's errors, are charged to the author. No page proofs are supplied.

Reprints

Order forms and a price list are sent with the proofs. Orders submitted after the issue is printed are subject to considerably higher prices.

KI09244

General Information

International Archives of
Allergy and Immunology

ISSN Print Edition: 1018–2438
ISSN Online Edition: 1423–0097

Journal Homepage: www.karger.com/iaa

Publication Data: 'International Archives of Allergy and Immunology' is published 12 times a year. Volumes 151–153, each with 4 issues, appear in 2010.

Subscription Rates: Subscriptions run for a full calendar year. Prices are given per year.

Personal subscription:

Print or Online	**Print+Online combined**
CHF 163.–	CHF 298.–
EUR 116.50	EUR 212.50
USD 155.00	USD 284.00

postage and handling (added to print and print+online)
CHF 75.60 Europe, CHF 113.40 Overseas
EUR 54.–
USD 107.40

Institutional subscription:

Print or Online	**Print+Online combined**
CHF 4446.–	CHF 4890.–
EUR 3177.–	EUR 3492.–
USD 4032.00	USD 4434.00

postage and handling (added to print and print+online)
CHF 94.80 Europe, CHF 141.60 Overseas
EUR 67.20
USD 134.40

Airmail surcharge: CHF 96.– / USD 91.20

Back Volumes and Single Issues: Information on availability and prices of single print issues and print or electronic back volumes can be obtained from Customer Service at *service@karger.ch.*

Bibliographic Indices: This journal is regularly listed in bibliographic services, including *Current Contents®* and PubMed/MEDLINE.

Subscription Orders:
Orders can be placed at agencies, bookstores, directly with the Publisher

S. Karger AG
Medical and Scientific Publishers
P.O. Box
CH–4009 Basel
Switzerland
(for courier services only:
Allschwilerstrasse 10
CH–4055 Basel)
Tel. +41 61 306 11 11
Fax +41 61 306 12 34
E-Mail karger@karger.ch
www.karger.com

or further Karger offices or representatives:

France:
Librairie Medi-Sciences Sarl
36, bd de Latour-Maubourg
75007 Paris
France
Tél. +33 1 45 51 42 58
Fax +33 1 45 56 07 80
E-Mail librairie@medi-sciences.fr
www.medi-sciences.fr

Germany:
S. Karger GmbH
Postfach
79095 Freiburg
Deutschland
(Hausadresse: Wilhelmstrasse 20 A
79098 Freiburg)
Tel. +49 761 45 20 70
Fax +49 761 45 20 714
E-Post information@karger.de
www.karger.de

India, Bangladesh, Sri Lanka:
Panther Publishers Private Ltd.
33, First Main
Koramangala First Block
Bangalore 560 034
India
Tel. +91 80 25505 836
Tel. +91 80 25505 837
Fax +91 80 25505 981
E-Mail panther_publishers@vsnl.com
www.pantherpublishers.com

Japan:
Karger Japan, Inc.
Yushima S Bld. 3F
4-2-3, Yushima, Bunkyo-ku
Tokyo 113-0034
Japan
Tel. +81 3 3815 1800
Fax +81 3 3815 1802
E-Mail publisher@karger.jp

China, Taiwan and Malaysia:
Karger China
Suite 409, Apollo Building
1440 Central Yan An Road
Shanghai 200040
China
Tel. +86 21 6133 1861
Fax +86 21 6133 1862
E-Mail karger.ray@gmail.com

South America and Central America:
Cranbury International LLC
7 Clarendon Ave., Suite 2
Montpelier, VT 05602
USA
Tel. +1 802 223 6565
Fax +1 802 223 6824
E-Mail
eatkin@cranburyinternational.com
www.cranburyinternational.com

United Kingdom, Ireland:
S. Karger AG
c/o London Liaison Office
4 Rickett Street
London SW6 1RU
United Kingdom
Tel. +44 20 7386 0500
Fax +44 20 7610 3337
E-Mail uk@karger.ch

USA:
S. Karger Publishers, Inc.
26 West Avon Road
P.O. Box 529
Unionville, CT 06085
USA
Toll free: +1 800 828 5479
Tel. +1 860 675 7834
Fax +1 860 675 7302
E-Mail karger@snet.net

Change of Address:
Both old and new address should be sent to the subscription source.

KARGER

Fax +41 61 306 12 34
E-Mail karger@karger.ch
www.karger.com

The Journal Home Page is available at:
www.karger.com/iaa

International Archives of
Allergy and Immunology

Eosinophils in Allergy and Related Diseases

Proceedings of a Workshop
Tokyo, Japan, June 20, 2009

Guest Editors
Takeshi Fukuda, Tochigi
Ken Ohta, Tokyo
Itsuo Iwamoto, Chiba
Takao Fujisawa, Mie
Akio Mori, Kanagawa
Junichi Chihara, Akita
Makoto Nagata, Saitama
Isao Ohno, Miyagi
Masahiko Kato, Gunma

47 figures, 3 in color, and 8 tables, 2010

KARGER
Basel · Freiburg · Paris · London · New York · Bangalore · Bangkok · Shanghai · Singapore · Tokyo · Sydney

Disclosure Statement Guest Editors

Takeshi Fukuda declares no conflict of interest.
Ken Ohta has received honoraria for lectures from GSK, AstraZeneca, Novartis, Merck, Schering-Plough, Teijin and Kyorin.
Itsuo Iwamoto declares no conflict of interest.
Takao Fujisawa declares no conflict of interest.
Akio Mori declares no conflict of interest.
Junichi Chihara declares no conflict of interest.
Makoto Nagato has received research grants to Saitama Medical University from AstraZeneca, GSK, Merck, Novartis, Schering-Plough and Teijin Pharma. He has received consulting fees from Astra-Zeneca, Boehringer-Ingelheim and Schering-Plough.
Isao Ohno declares no conflict of interest.
Masahiko Kato declares no conflict of interest.

S. Karger
Medical and Scientific Publishers
Basel • Freiburg • Paris • London • New York • Bangalore • Bangkok • Shanghai • Singapore • Tokyo • Sydney

Printed in Switzerland
on acid-free and non-aging paper (ISO 9706) by
Reinhardt Druck, Basel
ISBN 978–3–8055–9448–6
e-ISBN 978–3–8055–9449–3

KARGER

Fax +41 61 306 12 34
E-Mail karger@karger.ch
www.karger.com

Vol. 152, Suppl. 1, 2010

International Archives of
Allergy and
Immunology

Contents

KARGER

Fax +41 61 306 12 34
E-Mail karger@karger.ch
www.karger.com

Access to full text and tables of contents, including tentative ones for forthcoming issues: www.karger.com/iaa_issues

Reviews

International Archives of
Allergy and Immunology

Int Arch Allergy Immunol 2010;152(suppl 1):1
DOI: 10.1159/000312118

Published online: June 4, 2010

Preface

Since Paul Ehrlich discovered eosinophils in 1879, they have attracted significant interest since eosinophilia has been associated with allergy. Recent experimental and clinical advances in eosinophil-deficient mice and anti-interleukin-5 antibodies have improved our understanding of the role of eosinophils in the pathogenesis of allergic diseases such as asthma. Despite the growing body of information gained through research in cellular and molecular biology, we still do not know the precise roles of eosinophils in physiological conditions and/or in the cascade of events associated with eosinophilic disorders.

The 21st Annual Workshop on Eosinophils in Allergy and Related Diseases was held in Tokyo on June 20, 2009, with 21 cutting-edge research presentations. This workshop provided a forum for interested basic scientists and clinicians to exchange and discuss new insights regarding the role of eosinophils and other cells and factors involved in the pathogenesis of allergic diseases. I would like to thank all the participants who gave us the strength and energy to continue our research. I definitely believe that the talent of our membership will continue to promote excellence in future allergology research via mutual networking. It is our great pleasure to release the present proceedings, including peer-reviewed original papers and reviews. Several abstracts and titles which will be published in full elsewhere are also included.

The 6th Biennial International Symposium of the International Eosinophil Society was also held last year, in Bruges, Belgium. It was a great opportunity for scientists and clinicians/investigators from all over the world to meet, exchange information and spark collaborations to advance research in the fields of eosinophil-associated allergy and other diseases.

Finally, we would like to express our sincere gratitude to Novartis Pharma K.K. (Tokyo) for supporting this workshop, and to the staff of the International Medical Publishers Ltd. (Tokyo, Japan) for their excellent editing work.

Junichi Chihara, Akita, Japan

KARGER

Fax +41 61 306 12 34
E-Mail karger@karger.ch
www.karger.com

1018–2438/10/1525–0001$26.00/0

Accessible online at:
www.karger.com/iaa

Original Paper

International Archives of Allergy and Immunology

Int Arch Allergy Immunol 2010;152(suppl 1):2–8
DOI: 10.1159/000312119

Published online: June 4, 2010

Analysis of Signal Transduction Pathways Involved in Anti-CD30 mAb-Induced Human Eosinophil Apoptosis

Kenji Matsumoto[a] Maki Terakawa[a, b] Shuhei Fukuda[a] Hirohisa Saito[a]

[a]Department of Allergy and Immunology, National Research Institute for Child Health and Development, Tokyo, and [b]Asubio Pharma Co., Ltd., Osaka, Japan

Key Words

Apoptosis · CD30 · Eosinophils · Signal transduction pathways

Abstract

Background: Activation of cell surface CD30 by immobilized anti-CD30 monoclonal antibodies (mAbs) induces extremely rapid and intense apoptosis in human eosinophils in vitro. This anti-CD30 mAb-induced eosinophil apoptosis was inhibited by the addition of inhibitors of p38 and ERK1/2 mitogen-activated protein kinases (MAPKs). However, the signal transduction pathways other than for MAPKs remain unclear. In the present study, we tried to clarify the molecules involved in the induction of apoptosis after cross-linking of CD30. ***Methods:*** Purified human eosinophils were suspended in Iscove's minimal essential medium supplemented with 10% FCS and 1 ng/ml IL-5 and then cultured for 4 h in plates precoated with anti-CD30 mAb (clone Ber-H8) in the presence or absence of various signal transduction inhibitors. Eosinophil apoptosis was assessed using annexin V and flow cytometry. ***Results:*** The addition of inhibitors of caspase-3, caspase-8, pan-caspases, nuclear factor κB and protein kinase C at reasonable concentrations did not alter anti-CD30 mAb-induced eosinophil apoptosis in vitro. However, apoptosis was inhibited by phosphatidylinositol 3-kinase (PI3K) inhibitors: wortmannin at very high concentrations (>1 μM) significantly and LY294002 at a reasonable concentration partially inhibited that apoptosis. ***Conclusions:*** Anti-CD30 mAb-induced eosinophil apoptosis is likely to be mediated mainly through MAPKs and partially through PI3K, but independent of caspase activation. Downstream signaling molecules of MAPK activation in eosinophils have to be clarified in future studies.

Introduction

Eosinophils produce and release various kinds of cytokines, chemokines, granular proteins and other mediators in response to diverse physiological and artificial stimuli, and they play important roles in helminth infections and allergic diseases as both effector and modulatory cells [1–3]. Thus, one possible strategy for reducing allergic inflammation is to selectively induce apoptosis of eosinophils [4, 5]. An initial study using anti-IL-5 monoclonal antibody (mAb) failed to improve either allergic symptoms or airway hyperreactivity [6], suggesting that IL-5 is not crucial to eosinophil survival in lung tissue [7]. Subsequent studies proved that only half of lung-dwelling eosinophils were eliminated even after anti-IL-5 mAb

KARGER

Fax +41 61 306 12 34
E-Mail karger@karger.ch
www.karger.com

1018–2438/10/1525–0002$26.00/0

Accessible online at:
www.karger.com/iaa

Correspondence to: Dr. Kenji Matsumoto
Department of Allergy and Immunology
National Research Institute for Child Health and Development
2-10-1, Okura, Setagaya-ku, Tokyo 157-8535 (Japan)
Tel. +81 3 5494 7120, ext. 4955, Fax +81 3 5494 7028, E-Mail kmatsumoto@nch.go.jp

therapy and revealed that eosinophils play a critical role in airway remodeling in bronchial asthma [8, 9].

We previously demonstrated that immobilized anti-CD30 mAbs induced extremely rapid and intense apoptosis in human eosinophils in vitro [10]. We also demonstrated in vitro that anti-CD30 mAb-treated eosinophils are efficiently phagocytized by macrophages without releasing granular proteins [11].

CD30 was originally identified as Ki-1, an antigen expressed on Reed-Sternberg cells in Hodgkin's lymphoma [12]. Although numerous studies have attempted to elucidate the physiological and pathological roles of CD30, the actual roles of CD30 molecules in vivo remain obscure [13] even though a mouse CD30 knockout model was created [14]. CD30 is a member of the TNFR family, but unlike Fas and TRAIL receptors, it lacks an intracellular death domain [15]. Thus, it is of particular interest to reveal signal transduction pathways mediating eosinophil apoptosis via CD30. Using inhibitors of mitogen-activated protein kinases (MAPKs), we have already demonstrated that MAPKs play important roles in the induction of apoptosis [10]. However, other signal transduction pathways remain to be elucidated. In the present in vitro study, we tried to identify the molecules involved in the induction of apoptosis in human eosinophils after cross-linking of CD30.

Materials and Methods

mAbs and Reagents

Two different clones of apoptosis-inducing anti-CD30 mAbs and a clone of a non-apoptosis-inducing anti-CD30 mAb were obtained from the indicated sources: clone HRS-4 (IgG1, Immunotech, Marseilles, France), clone Ber-H8 (IgG1, Pharmingen, San Diego, Calif., USA) and clone Ber-H2 (IgG1, Dako, Glostrup, Denmark). An isotype-matched irrelevant control mAb (IgG1, MOPC-21) was purchased from Sigma (St. Louis, Mo., USA). When necessary, mAbs were dialyzed against PBS (Sigma) to remove NaN_3 prior to use. Specific inhibitors of caspase-3 (z-DEVD-fmk), caspase-8 (z-IETD-fmk) and pan-caspases (z-VAD-fmk) were obtained from the Medical Biological Laboratory (Nagoya, Japan). The following inhibitors of signal transduction pathways were obtained from Calbiochem, San Diego, Calif., USA: nuclear factor (NF)-κB inhibitors, MG-132 and SN50; a protein kinase C (PKC) inhibitor, staurosporine, and a phosphatidylinositol 3-kinase (PI3K) inhibitor, wortmannin.

Eosinophil Preparation

Eosinophils were purified from the peripheral blood of normal subjects and subjects with mild allergic diseases (n = 12) by Ficoll-sodium diatrizoate density gradient (Lymphocyte Separation Medium; MP Biomedicals, Aurora, Ohio, USA) sedimentation and negative selection with anti-CD16 antibody-coated immunomagnetic beads (Miltenyi Biotec, Bergisch Gladbach, Germany), as previously described [16]. Both the purity and viability of the eosinophils were confirmed to exceed 99% based on light-microscopic examination of cytocentrifuged preparations stained with Diff-Quik (American Scientific Products, McGraw Park, Ill., USA) and by trypan blue dye (Sigma) exclusion, respectively. All the allergic donors were diagnosed as having either allergic rhinitis and/or bronchial asthma, but they had no more than mild symptoms at the time of blood collection. Written informed consent was obtained from all subjects, and the study was approved by the Ethical Review Board of the National Research Institute for Child Health and Development, Tokyo, Japan.

Eosinophil Culture and Survival Assay

Purified eosinophils were suspended at a cell density of 1×10^6/ml in Iscove's modified Dulbecco's medium (Gibco, Grand Island, N.Y., USA) supplemented with 10% FCS (HyClone Laboratories, Logan, Utah, USA) and 1 ng/ml IL-5 (R&D Systems, Minneapolis, Minn., USA). The cells were then cultured in 24-well culture plates (Costar, Cambridge, Mass., USA) precoated with 10 μg/ml of either anti-CD30 mAb or control IgG1 overnight at 4°C in the presence or absence of various signal transduction inhibitors.

Cell viability was examined with an apoptosis detection kit (MEBCYTO-Apoptosis Kit; Medical Biological Laboratories, Nagoya, Japan) using FITC-conjugated annexin V [17] and propidium iodide (PI) according to the manufacturers' instructions. Briefly, after 4 h of incubation, cultured eosinophils were harvested by gentle pipetting and washed once with PBS. The harvested eosinophils were then suspended in a Ca^{2+}-containing buffer and reacted with FITC-conjugated annexin V for 15 min at room temperature. One minute before flow-cytometric analysis (FACS Calibur; Becton-Dickinson, Mountain View, Calif., USA), the eosinophils were also stained with 10 μg/ml PI. The FITC-stained cells (annexin V positive) and PI-stained cells were assessed by flow cytometry as previously described [10]. All culture experiments were performed in duplicate.

Statistical Analysis

All the data are presented as means ± SEM unless otherwise indicated. Differences between groups were analyzed using the paired t test and considered to be significant at $p < 0.05$.

Results

Effects of Caspase Inhibitors on Anti-CD30 mAb-Induced Eosinophil Apoptosis

Eosinophils were cultured in either anti-CD30 mAb (HRS-4, Ber-H2 or Ber-H8)- or IgG1 control mAb-coated plates for 4 h (fig. 1). Annexin V-positive eosinophils were determined by flow cytometry. The rate of annexin V positivity was significantly higher in the eosinophils cultured in the HRS-4 and Ber-H8 anti-CD30 mAbs-coated plates than in the eosinophils cultured in either the anti-CD30 mAb (Ber-H2)-coated or irrelevant control IgG1-coated plates ($p < 0.05$). These results

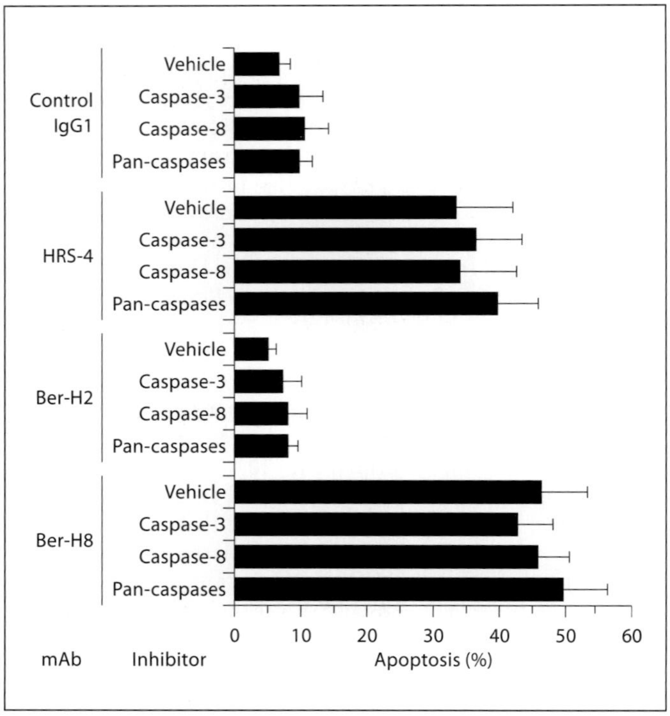

Fig. 1. Effects of caspase inhibitors on anti-CD30 mAb-induced eosinophil apoptosis. Purified eosinophils were cultured in either 10 μg/ml anti-CD30 mAb (HRS-4, Ber-H8 or Ber-H2)- or IgG1 control mAb-coated plates for 4 h in the presence or absence of 20 μg/ml of inhibitors of caspase-3, caspase-8 and pan-caspases. Annexin V-positive eosinophils were measured by flow cytometry. Means ± SEM of 3 separate experiments from 3 different donors performed in duplicate.

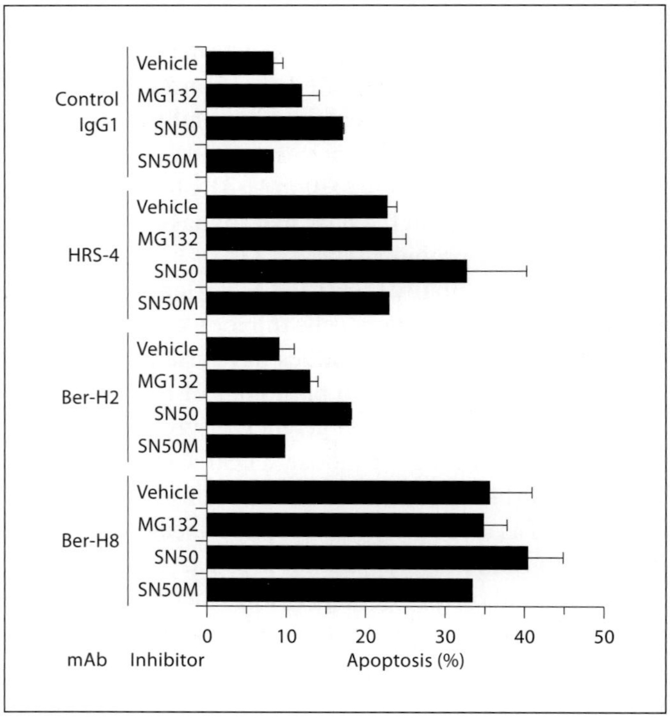

Fig. 2. Effects of NF-κB inhibitors on anti-CD30 mAb-induced eosinophil apoptosis. Purified eosinophils were cultured in either 10 μg/ml anti-CD30 mAb (HRS-4, Ber-H8 or Ber-H2)- or IgG1 control mAb-coated plates for 4 h in the presence or absence of 100 μM MG-132, 100 μM SN50 or 100 μM SN50M (negative control of SN50). Annexin V-positive eosinophils were measured by flow cytometry. Means ± SEM of 3 separate experiments from 3 different donors performed in duplicate.

are compatible with the results obtained in our previous study [10].

To determine the involvement of caspases in this apoptosis, two different concentrations of specific inhibitors of different caspases were added. Addition of 20 μM of specific inhibitors of caspase-3, caspase-8 and pan-caspases showed no effects on anti-CD30 mAb (HRS-4 and Ber-H8)-induced eosinophil apoptosis (fig. 1). These three inhibitors also had no effects on anti-CD30 mAb (HRS-4 and Ber-H8)-induced eosinophil apoptosis even at concentrations as high as 200 μM (data not shown).

Effects of NF-κB Inhibitors on Anti-CD30 mAb-Induced Eosinophil Apoptosis

Eosinophils were cultured in either anti-CD30 mAb (HRS-4, Ber-H2 or Ber-H8)- or IgG1 control mAb-coated plates for 4 h in the presence or absence of 10 or 100 μM of MG-132, SN50 or SN50M (negative control of SN50). The addition of MG132 and SN50M at any concentration showed no effects on anti-CD30 mAb (HRS-4 and Ber-H8)-induced eosinophil apoptosis (fig. 2). SN50 at 100 μM significantly enhanced spontaneous eosinophil apoptosis (eosinophils cultured in plates coated with control IgG1 or Ber-H2) and showed a slight tendency to enhance anti-CD30 mAb (HRS-4 and Ber-H8)-induced eosinophil apoptosis. However, at 10 μM, SN50 showed absolutely no effect on eosinophil apoptosis (data not shown).

Effect of PKC Inhibitor on the Anti-CD30 mAb-Induced Eosinophil Apoptosis

Eosinophils were cultured in either anti-CD30 mAb (Ber-H8)- or IgG1 control mAb-coated plates for 4 h in the presence or absence of various concentrations of staurosporine (fig. 3a). Staurosporine at up to 10 μM showed no effect on anti-CD30 mAb (Ber-H8)-induced eosinophil apoptosis. Next, the highest concentration (10 μM) of staurosporine was added to eosinophils cultured in either anti-CD30 mAb (HRS-4, Ber-H2 or Ber-H8)- or

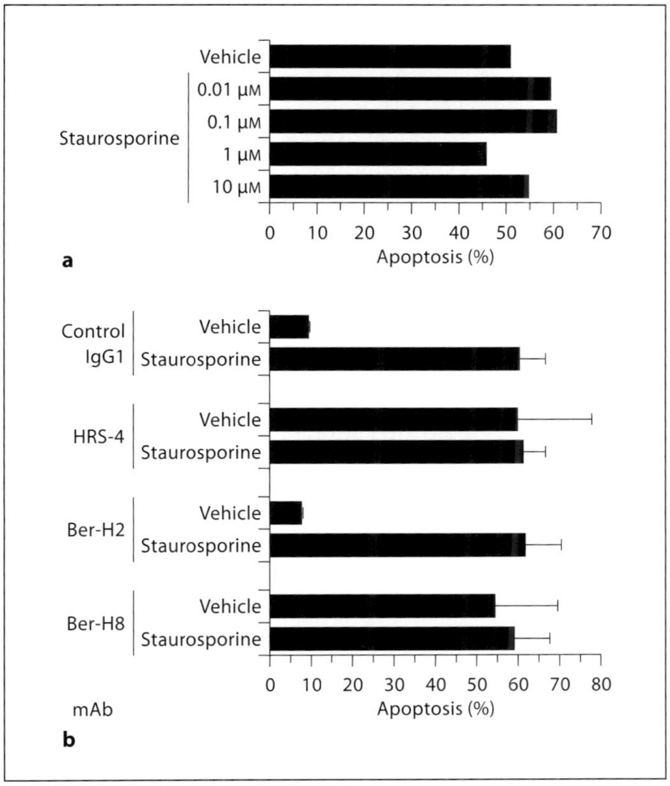

Fig. 3. Effect of a PKC inhibitor on anti-CD30 mAb-induced eosinophil apoptosis. **a** Purified eosinophils were cultured in 10 μg/ml anti-CD30 mAb (Ber-H8)-coated plates for 4 h in the presence or absence of various concentrations of staurosporine. Annexin V-positive eosinophils were measured by flow cytometry. Values represent the mean of duplicates representative of 2 separate experiments from 2 different donors. **b** Purified eosinophils were cultured in either 10 μg/ml anti-CD30 mAb (HRS-4, Ber-H8 or Ber-H2)- or IgG1 control mAb-coated plates for 4 h in the presence or absence of 10 μM staurosporine. Annexin V-positive eosinophils were measured by flow cytometry. Means ± SEM of 3 separate experiments from 3 different donors performed in duplicate.

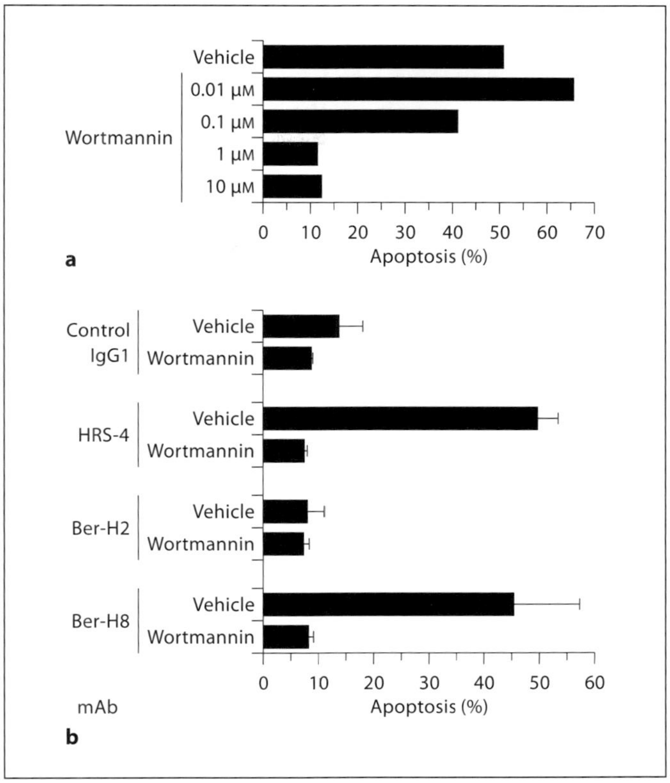

Fig. 4. Effect of a PI3K inhibitor on anti-CD30 mAb-induced eosinophil apoptosis. **a** Purified eosinophils were cultured in 10 μg/ml anti-CD30 mAb (Ber-H8)-coated plates for 4 h in the presence or absence of various concentrations of wortmannin. Annexin V-positive eosinophils were measured by flow cytometry. Values represent the mean of duplicates representative of 2 separate experiments for 2 different donors. **b** Purified eosinophils were cultured in either 10 μg/ml anti-CD30 mAb (HRS-4, Ber-H8 or Ber-H2)- or IgG1 control mAb-coated plates for 4 h in the presence or absence of 10 μM wortmannin. Annexin V-positive eosinophils were measured by flow cytometry. Means ± SEM of 3 separate experiments from 3 different donors performed in duplicate.

IgG1 control mAb-coated plates for 4 h, and eosinophil viability was evaluated (fig. 3b). Again, 10 μM staurosporine did not affect anti-CD30 mAb (HRS-4 and Ber-H8)-induced eosinophil apoptosis. In contrast, staurosporine significantly enhanced spontaneous eosinophil apoptosis (eosinophils cultured in plates coated with control IgG1 or Ber-H2).

Effect of PI3K Inhibitor on the Anti-CD30 mAb-Induced Eosinophil Apoptosis

Eosinophils were cultured in either anti-CD30 mAb (Ber-H8)- or IgG1 control mAb-coated plates for 4 h in the presence or absence of various concentrations of wortmannin (fig. 4a). Wortmannin at up to 0.1 μM showed no effect on anti-CD30 mAb (Ber-H8)-induced eosinophil apoptosis, but 1 and 10 μM wortmannin significantly inhibited apoptosis. Next, the highest concentration (10 μM) of wortmannin was added to eosinophils cultured in anti-CD30 mAb (HRS-4, Ber-H2 or Ber-H8)- or IgG1 control mAb-coated plates for 4 h, and eosinophil viability was measured (fig. 4b). Again, the addition of 10 μM wortmannin resulted in significant inhibition of anti-CD30 mAb (HRS-4 and Ber-H8)-induced eosinophil apoptosis. In contrast, wortmannin did not alter spontaneous eosinophil apoptosis (eosinophils cultured in plates coated with control IgG1 or Ber-H2).

Discussion

To date, several surface molecules, including Fas [18], CD69 [19], CD45RA [20] and Siglec 8 [21], have been shown to be capable of inducing apoptosis in eosinophils. Among these molecules, CD30 induces the most rapid and intense apoptosis of eosinophils in vitro [10]. However, this effect was only seen when the anti-CD30 mAbs were immobilized, not in soluble form, suggesting that cross-linking of cell surface CD30 or a second signal is essential for the induction of this apoptosis [10]. In addition, the fact that not all mAbs against CD30 induce apoptosis in eosinophils suggests involvement of some specific signal transduction pathway(s) [10].

Recently, several signal transduction pathway molecules related to cell survival, including caspases [22, 23], NF-κB [23], PKC [24], PI3K [25] and MAPKs [26–28], have been shown to be activated upon stimulation via CD30 in other cell types. To clarify the apoptosis signal transduction pathway via CD30 in eosinophils is nonetheless important because the molecules involved may serve as new potential targets for regulating eosinophil survival. Thus, we tried to elucidate the involvement of all signal transduction pathways known to be activated after cross-linking of CD30.

First, we examined whether caspases are involved in the signal transduction pathways in eosinophil apoptosis after anti-CD30 mAb treatment. As shown in figure 1, specific inhibitors of caspase-3 (IC_{50} = 5 μM) [29], caspase-8 (IC_{50} = 5 μM) [30] and even pan-caspases (IC_{50} = 5 μM) [29] at up to 200 μM showed no effect on anti-CD30 mAb (HRS-4 and Ber-H8)-induced eosinophil apoptosis. This result was compatible with the fact that CD30 lacks an intracellular death domain capable of activating caspase-3 directly [15].

Next, we examined whether NF-κB, a well-known molecule that is activated upon cross-linking of most TNFR family members [15], is involved in the signal transduction pathways in eosinophil apoptosis. We found that an NF-κB inhibitor, MG-132 (IC_{50} = 3 μM) [31], at up to 100 μM showed no effect on anti-CD30 mAb (HRS-4 and Ber-H8)-induced eosinophil apoptosis (fig. 2). Another NF-κB-specific inhibitor, SN50 (IC_{50} = 11 μM) [32] at 100 μM, but not its negative control, SN50M, showed a tendency to enhance not only spontaneous but also anti-CD30 mAb (HRS-4 and Ber-H8)-induced eosinophil apoptosis (fig. 2), suggesting that NF-κB signaling is not involved in the induction of eosinophil apoptosis via CD30.

Then we examined whether PKC is involved in the signal transduction pathways in eosinophil apoptosis after anti-CD30 mAb treatment [33]. Staurosporine inhibits a wide range of protein kinases, including PKC (IC_{50} = 0.7 nM), protein kinase A (IC_{50} = 7 nM), protein kinase G (IC_{50} = 8.5 nM), myosin light-chain kinase (IC_{50} = 1.3 nM) and CaM kinase (IC_{50} = 20 nM). As shown in figure 3a, regardless of the concentration of staurosporine, anti-CD30 mAb (Ber-H8)-induced eosinophil apoptosis was not altered. A similar result was also obtained when another PKC inhibitor, bisindolylmaleimide, was used (data not shown). In contrast, a very high concentration (>100 nM) of staurosporine was shown to rapidly activate the mitochondrial-mediated apoptotic pathway in several cell lines [34]. In our experiments, a very high concentration (10 μM) of staurosporine actually induced eosinophil apoptosis regardless of anti-CD30 mAb treatment (fig. 3b). These data strongly suggest that PKC is unlikely to be involved in the signal transduction pathways for induction of eosinophil apoptosis via CD30.

Finally, to examine whether PI3K is involved in the signal transduction pathways in eosinophil apoptosis after anti-CD30 mAb treatment [35], we added different concentrations of wortmannin to the anti-CD30 mAb-induced eosinophil apoptosis assay. Wortmannin is a well-known inhibitor of PI3K at a low concentration (IC_{50} = 5 nM), while it also inhibits MAPK, especially Ca^{2+}-independent MAPKs at a very high concentration (>0.5 μM) [36]. We found that low concentrations of wortmannin did not affect anti-CD30 mAb (Ber-H8)-induced eosinophil apoptosis (fig. 4a). However, higher concentrations (>1 μM) of wortmannin significantly inhibited anti-CD30 mAb (Ber-H8)-induced eosinophil apoptosis in vitro (fig. 4a); 10 μM wortmannin completely abrogated apoptosis induction via CD30 (fig. 4b). In addition, another specific inhibitor of PI3K, LY294002, at a reasonable concentration partially inhibited that apoptosis (data not shown). These data suggest that anti-CD30 mAb-induced eosinophil apoptosis is likely to be mediated mainly through MAPKs and partially through PI3K. This result was compatible with our previous report that inhibitors of two types of MAPKs, p38 and ERK1/2, block anti-CD30 mAb-induced eosinophil apoptosis in a dose-dependent manner [10]. Addition of different concentrations of a calcium-chelating reagent [1,2-bis(*o*-aminophenoxy)ethane-N,N,N′,N′-tetraacetic acid] showed absolutely no effect on this apoptosis (data not shown), suggesting that MAPKs involved in this signal transduction pathway are Ca^{2+} independent.

With respect to the results of our previous study [10] and our present experiments, especially those obtained using a very high concentration of wortmannin, MAPKs are critically involved in anti-CD30 mAb-induced eosinophil apoptosis in vitro, whereas caspase activation is unlikely to be involved. Downstream signaling molecules of MAPK activation in eosinophils remain to be clarified in future studies.

Acknowledgment

This work was supported in part by a grant from the Ministry of Education, Culture, Sports, Science and Technology (No. 20591196 to K.M.).

Disclosure Statement

M.T. is employed by Asubio Pharma Co., Ltd. The rest of the authors declare that no financial or other conflict of interest exists in relation to the content of this article.

References

1 Kay AB, Phipps S, Robinson DS: A role for eosinophils in airway remodelling in asthma. Trends Immunol 2004;25:477–482.
2 Gomes I, Mathur SK, Espenshade BM, Mori Y, Varga J, Ackerman SJ: Eosinophil-fibroblast interactions induce fibroblast IL-6 secretion and extracellular matrix gene expression: implications in fibrogenesis. J Allergy Clin Immunol 2005;116:796–804.
3 Rothenberg ME, Hogan SP: The eosinophil. Annu Rev Immunol 2006;24:147–174.
4 Ying S, Meng Q, Taborda-Barata L, Kay AB: Association of apoptosis of neutrophils and eosinophils and their ingestion by macrophages with resolution of the allergen-induced cutaneous late-phase response in atopic human subjects. Proc Assoc Am Physicians 1997;109:42–50.
5 Haslett C: Granulocyte apoptosis and its role in the resolution and control of lung inflammation. Am J Respir Crit Care Med 1999; 160:S5–S11.
6 Leckie MJ, ten Brinke A, Khan J, Diamant Z, O'Connor BJ, Walls CM, Mathur AK, Cowley HC, Chung KF, Djukanovic R, Hansel TT, Holgate ST, Sterk PJ, Barnes PJ: Effects of an interleukin-5 blocking monoclonal antibody on eosinophils, airway hyper-responsiveness, and the late asthmatic response. Lancet 2000;356:2144–2148.
7 Liu LY, Sedgwick JB, Bates ME, Vrtis RF, Gern JE, Kita H, Jarjour NN, Busse WW, Kelly EA: Decreased expression of membrane IL-5 receptor alpha on human eosinophils: I. Loss of membrane IL-5 receptor alpha on airway eosinophils and increased soluble IL-5 receptor alpha in the airway after allergen challenge. J Immunol 2002;169: 6452–6458.
8 Flood-Page P, Menzies-Gow A, Phipps S, Ying S, Wangoo A, Ludwig MS, Barnes N, Robinson D, Kay AB: Anti-IL-5 treatment reduces deposition of ECM proteins in the bronchial subepithelial basement membrane of mild atopic asthmatics. J Clin Invest 2003; 112:1029–1036.
9 Broide DH: Immunologic and inflammatory mechanisms that drive asthma progression to remodeling. J Allergy Clin Immunol 2008; 121:560–570.
10 Matsumoto K, Terakawa M, Miura K, Fukuda S, Nakajima T, Saito H: Extremely rapid and intense induction of apoptosis in human eosinophils by anti-CD30 antibody treatment in vitro. J Immunol 2004;172:2186–2193.
11 Matsumoto K, Terakawa M, Fukuda S, Saito H: Rapid and strong induction of apoptosis in human eosinophils by anti-CD30 mAb-coated microspheres and phagocytosis by macrophages. Int Arch Allergy Immunol 2007;143(suppl 1):60–67.
12 Dürkop H, Latza U, Hummel M, Eitelbach F, Seed B, Stein H: Molecular cloning and expression of a new member of the nerve growth factor receptor family that is characteristic for Hodgkin's disease. Cell 1992;68: 421–427.
13 Horie R, Watanabe T: CD30: expression and function in health and disease. Semin Immunol 1998;10:457–470.
14 Amakawa R, Hakem A, Kundig TM, Matsuyama T, Simard JJ, Timms E, Wakeham A, Mittruecker HW, Griesser H, Takimoto H, Schmits R, Shahinian A, Ohashi P, Penninger JM, Mak TW: Impaired negative selection of T cells in Hodgkin's disease antigen CD30-deficient mice. Cell 1996;84: 551–562.
15 Watts TH: TNF/TNFR family members in costimulation of T cell responses. Annu Rev Immunol 2005;23:23–68.
16 Hansel TT, De VI, Iff T, Rihs S, Wandzilak M, Betz S, Blaser K, Walker C: An improved immunomagnetic procedure for the isolation of highly purified human blood eosinophils. J Immunol Methods 1991;145:105–110.
17 Vermes I, Haanen C, Steffens-Nakken H, Reutelingsperger C: A novel assay for apoptosis. Flow cytometric detection of phosphatidylserine expression on early apoptotic cells using fluorescein labelled annexin V. J Immunol Methods 1995;184:39–51.
18 Matsumoto K, Schleimer RP, Saito H, Iikura Y, Bochner BS: Induction of apoptosis in human eosinophils by anti-Fas antibody treatment in vitro. Blood 1995;86:1437–1443.
19 Walsh GM, Williamson ML, Symon FA, Willars GB, Wardlaw AJ: Ligation of CD69 induces apoptosis and cell death in human eosinophils cultured with granulocyte-macrophage colony-stimulating factor. Blood 1996;87:2815–2821.
20 Blaylock MG, Sexton DW, Walsh GM: Ligation of CD45 and the isoforms CD45RA and CD45RB accelerates the rate of constitutive apoptosis in human eosinophils. J Allergy Clin Immunol 1999;104:1244–1250.
21 Nutku E, Aizawa H, Hudson SA, Bochner BS: Ligation of Siglec-8: a selective mechanism for induction of human eosinophil apoptosis. Blood 2003;101:5014–5020.
22 Clarke LE, Bayerl MG, Bruggeman RD, Mauger D, Ioffreda MD, Abou-Elella A, Helm KF: Death receptor apoptosis signaling mediated by FADD in CD30-positive lymphoproliferative disorders involving the skin. Am J Surg Pathol 2005;29:452–459.
23 Hirsch B, Hummel M, Bentink S, Fouladi F, Spang R, Zollinger R, Stein H, Durkop H: CD30-induced signaling is absent in Hodgkin's cells but present in anaplastic large cell lymphoma cells. Am J Pathol 2008;172:510–520.
24 Nery FC, Passos DO, Garcia VS, Kobarg J: Ki-1/57 interacts with RACK1 and is a substrate for the phosphorylation by phorbol 12-myristate 13-acetate-activated protein kinase C. J Biol Chem 2004;279:11444–11455.
25 Georgakis GV, Li Y, Rassidakis GZ, Medeiros LJ, Mills GB, Younes A: Inhibition of the phosphatidylinositol-3 kinase/Akt promotes G1 cell cycle arrest and apoptosis in Hodgkin lymphoma. Br J Haematol 2006; 132:503–511.

26 Wendtner CM, Schmitt B, Gruss HJ, Druker BJ, Emmerich B, Goodwin RG, Hallek M: CD30 ligand signal transduction involves activation of a tyrosine kinase and of mitogen-activated protein kinase in a Hodgkin's lymphoma cell line. Cancer Res 1995;55: 4157–4161.

27 Schneider C, Stohr D, Merz H, Hubinger G: Signal transduction in anaplastic large cell lymphoma cells (ALCL) mediated by the tumor necrosis factor receptor CD30. Leuk Lymphoma 2004;45:1009–1015.

28 Krysov SV, Rowley TF, Al-Shamkhani A: Inhibition of p38 mitogen-activated protein kinase unmasks a CD30-triggered apoptotic pathway in anaplastic large cell lymphoma cells. Mol Cancer Ther 2007;6:703–711.

29 Atkinson EA, Barry M, Darmon AJ, Shostak I, Turner PC, Moyer RW, Bleackley RC: Cytotoxic T lymphocyte-assisted suicide. Caspase 3 activation is primarily the result of the direct action of granzyme B. J Biol Chem 1998;273:21261–21266.

30 Kobayashi T, Okamoto K, Kobata T, Hasunuma T, Sumida T, Nishioka K: Tumor necrosis factor alpha regulation of the FAS-mediated apoptosis-signaling pathway in synovial cells. Arthritis Rheum 1999;42: 519–526.

31 Adams J, Stein R: Novel inhibitors of the proteasome and their therapeutic use in inflammation. Annu Rep Med Chem 1996;31:279–288.

32 Lin YZ, Yao SY, Veach RA, Torgerson TR, Hawiger J: Inhibition of nuclear translocation of transcription factor NF-kappa B by a synthetic peptide containing a cell membrane-permeable motif and nuclear localization sequence. J Biol Chem 1995;270:14255–14258.

33 Cousin JM, Haslett C, Rossi AG: Regulation of granulocyte apoptosis by PKC inhibition and elevation of [Ca2+]i. Biochem Soc Trans 1997;25:243S.

34 Widenmaier SB, Ao Z, Kim SJ, Warnock G, McIntosh CH: Suppression of p38 MAPK and JNK via Akt-mediated inhibition of apoptosis signal-regulating kinase 1 constitutes a core component of the beta-cell pro-survival effects of glucose-dependent insulinotropic polypeptide. J Biol Chem 2009;30; 284:30372–30382.

35 Pinho V, Souza DG, Barsante MM, Hamer FP, De Freitas MS, Rossi AG, Teixeira MM: Phosphoinositide-3 kinases critically regulate the recruitment and survival of eosinophils in vivo: importance for the resolution of allergic inflammation. J Leukoc Biol 2005; 77:800–810.

36 Ferby I, Waga I, Kume K, Sakanaka C, Shimizu T: PAF-induced MAPK activation is inhibited by wortmannin in neutrophils and macrophages. Adv Exp Med Biol 1996;416: 321–326.

Original Paper

International Archives of Allergy and Immunology

Int Arch Allergy Immunol 2010;152(suppl 1):9–17
DOI: 10.1159/000312120

Published online: June 4, 2010

Cooperative Activation of CCL5 Expression by TLR3 and Tumor Necrosis Factor-α or Interferon-γ through Nuclear Factor-κB or STAT-1 in Airway Epithelial Cells

Tetsuya Homma[a] Satoshi Matsukura[a] Takashi Hirose[a] Tsukasa Ohnishi[a] Teruaki Kimura[a] Masatsugu Kurokawa[a] Koushi Ieki[a] Miho Odaka[a] Shintaro Suzuki[a] Shin Watanabe[a] Masayuki Sato[a] Mio Kawaguchi[b] Robert P. Schleimer[c] Mitsuru Adachi[a]

[a]Division of Respiratory Medicine and Allergy, Department of Internal Medicine, Showa University School of Medicine, Tokyo, and [b]Department of Respiratory Medicine, Institute of Clinical Medicine, University of Tsukuba, Tsukuba, Japan; [c]Division of Allergy and Immunology, Northwestern University Feinberg School of Medicine, Chicago, Ill., USA

Key Words

Airway epithelial cells · CCL5/RANTES · Nuclear factor-κB · STAT-1 · TLR3

Abstract

Background: CCL5/RANTES contributes to prolonged eosinophilic inflammation and asthma exacerbation after a viral infection. We studied the mechanism of CCL5 expression using viral product double-stranded RNA (dsRNA), a ligand of Toll-like receptor 3 (TLR3), and inflammatory cytokines in airway epithelial cells. ***Methods:*** The airway epithelial cell line BEAS-2B was used in our in vitro study, and the levels of CCL5 mRNA and CCL5 protein expression were determined using real-time PCR and ELISA. The activity of the CCL5 promoter region and nuclear factor (NF)-κB was assessed by dual luciferase assay using specific luciferase reporter plasmids. We used actinomycin D to assess the stability of mRNA. Phosphorylation of signal transducer and activator of transcription 1 (STAT-1) was analyzed by Western blot. ***Results:*** Synthetic dsRNA up-regulated the expression of CCL5 mRNA and CCL5 protein. Adding TNF-α or IFN-γ to dsRNA further increased the expression of CCL5. The combination of TNF-α and dsRNA cooperatively activated the CCL5 promoter region and the NF-κB-specific reporter. IFN-γ did not activate these reporters. However, it increased the stability of CCL5 mRNA induced by dsRNA. IFN-γ phosphorylated STAT-1, but dsRNA did not. The effects of IFN-γ were not evident in the cells transfected with short interfering RNA for STAT-1. ***Conclusions:*** Cross-talk between TLR3 signaling and inflammatory cytokines regulates the expression of CCL5 in airway epithelial cells. In this mechanism, TNF-α may activate NF-κB, in cooperation with TLR3 signaling. IFN-γ may stabilize CCL5 mRNA up-regulated by TLR3. This mechanism may depend on STAT-1.

Introduction

CCL5/RANTES is a chemokine that attracts inflammatory cells, including eosinophils, into the airways. Its up-regulation in airway epithelial cells may contribute to prolonged eosinophilic inflammation and asthma exac-

KARGER

Fax +41 61 306 12 34
E-Mail karger@karger.ch
www.karger.com

1018–2438/10/1525–0009$26.00/0

Accessible online at:
www.karger.com/iaa

Correspondence to: Dr. Satoshi Matsukura
Division of Respiratory Medicine and Allergy, Department of Internal Medicine
Showa University School of Medicine
1-5-8 Hatanodai, Shinagawa-ku, Tokyo 142-8666 (Japan)
Tel. +81 3 3784 8532, Fax +81 3 3784 8742, E-Mail smatsuku@med.showa-u.ac.jp

erbation after an infection by viruses, such as the human rhinovirus, respiratory syncytial virus and influenza viruses [1–3].

TNF-α and IFN-γ are cytokines produced by macrophages, lymphocytes and dendritic cells during a viral infection. These cytokines are important for innate immunity against viruses. On the other hand, TNF-α or IFN-γ stimulates airway inflammation and prolong asthma exacerbation after a viral infection [4, 5]. Viruses such as human rhinovirus, respiratory syncytial virus and influenza viruses up-regulate the expression of CCL5. TNF-α and IFN-γ enhance CCL5 expression [6–10]. The mechanisms of the cooperative activation of viruses and cytokines are not fully understood.

We previously reported that double-stranded RNA (dsRNA) activates CCL5 expression, which is mediated through the Toll-like receptor 3 (TLR3) in airway epithelial cells. The activation of CCL5 transcription by dsRNA depends on the presence of the transcription factor nuclear factor (NF)-κB and interferon regulatory factor 3 (IRF-3) [11–13]. In this study, we hypothesize that inflammatory cytokines such as TNF-α or IFN-γ may stimulate TLR3 signaling and activate CCL5 expression in airway epithelial cells. We also focused on the mechanisms of the cooperative activation of CCL5 expression by TLR3 and either TNF-α or IFN-γ.

Material and Methods

Cell Culture and Reagents

BEAS-2B is a human airway epithelial cell line transformed with an adenovirus 12-SV40 virus hybrid that we purchased from American Type Culture Collection. BEAS-2B cells were cultured in DMEM/F12 with 10% FBS, 100 U/ml penicillin and 100 ng/ml streptomycin (Invitrogen, Tokyo, Japan) at 37°C with 5% CO_2 in humidified air and were treated as described previously [12]. We purchased synthetic dsRNA polyinosinic:polycytidylic acid (poly I:C) from Sigma (Tokyo, Japan) and recombinant human TNF-α and IFN-γ from R&D Systems (Tokyo, Japan).

Real-Time PCR

Purification of RNA and synthesis of cDNA was performed as described previously [12]. A pre-designed TaqMan probe set for CCL5 mRNA was obtained from Applied Biosystems (Tokyo, Japan). Each probe has a fluorescent reporter dye (FAM) linked to its 5′ end and a downstream quencher dye (TAMRA) linked to its 3′ end. We used TaqMan ribosomal RNA probe, which is labeled with a fluorescent reporter dye (VIC), as an internal control. Each reaction consisted of 25 μl containing 2× Universal Master Mix (Applied Biosystems), primers, labeled probes and 50 ng cDNA. Amplification conditions consisted of 40 cycles at 95°C for 15 s and 60°C for 1 min after incubation with 95°C for 10 min. Amplification and fluorescent measurements were carried out during the elongation step with an ABI PRISM 7700 Sequence Detection System (Applied Biosystems). Data are shown as fold induction of non-stimulated control cells [12].

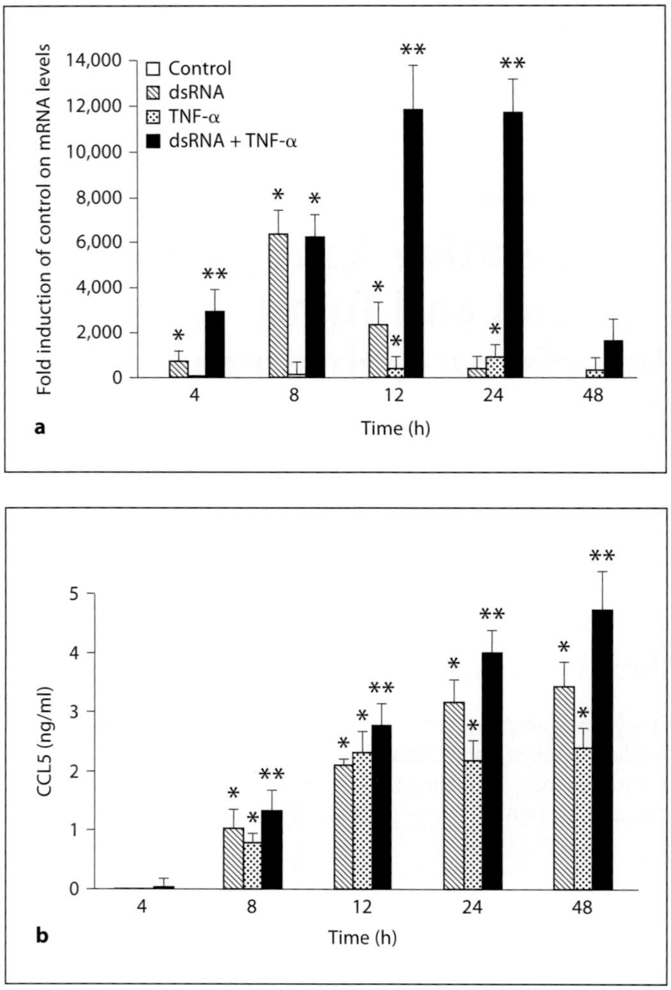

Fig. 1. Effect of TNF-α plus dsRNA on CCL5 mRNA expression (**a**) and protein release into the media (**b**). The BEAS-2B cells were incubated with synthetic dsRNA poly I:C (10 μg/ml) and/or TNF-α (10 ng/ml) for 4–48 h prior to real-time PCR or ELISA. Means ± SEM of three independent experiments. * $p < 0.05$ vs. non-stimulated control cells at the same time point; ** $p < 0.05$ vs. cells stimulated with dsRNA at the same time point.

Assay of CCL5 Release into the Culture Medium

The concentration of CCL5 in collected cell culture media was assessed using a commercially available enzyme-linked immunosorbent assay (ELISA) kit (R&D Systems, Tokyo, Japan), as described previously [11, 12].

Transient Transfections and Luciferase Assay

To investigate transcriptional mechanisms, we used firefly-luciferase reporter vectors (a kind gift from Dr. Tomas J. Schall)

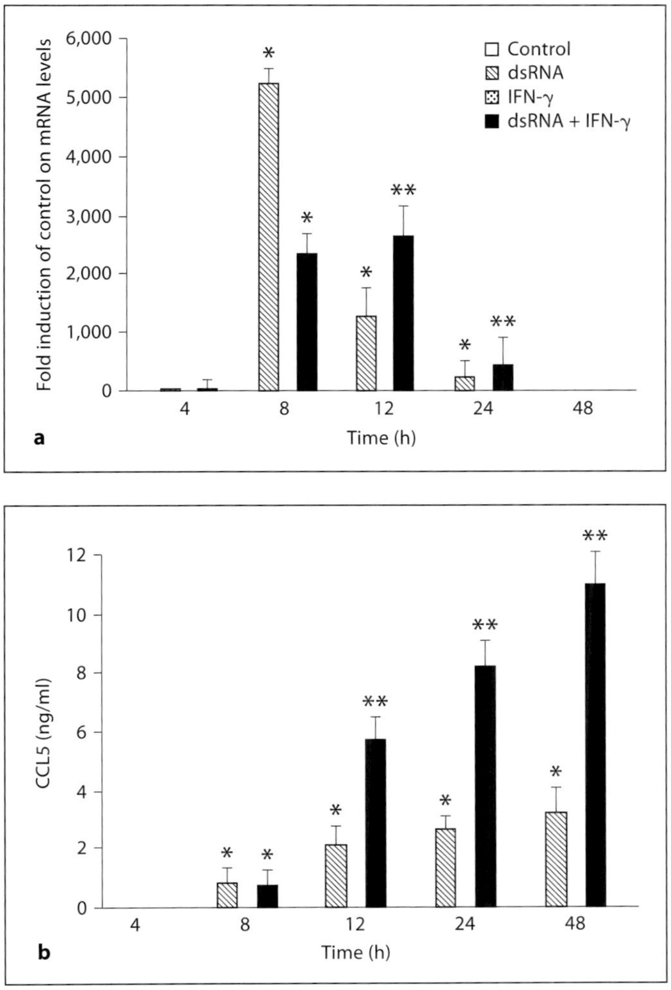

Fig. 2. Effect of IFN-γ plus dsRNA on CCL5 mRNA expression (**a**) and protein release into the media (**b**). BEAS-2B cells were incubated with synthetic dsRNA poly I:C (10 μg/ml) and/or IFN-γ (50 ng/ml) for 4–48 h prior to real-time PCR or ELISA. Means ± SEM of three independent experiments. * $p < 0.05$ vs. non-stimulated control cells at the same time point; ** $p < 0.05$ vs. cells stimulated with dsRNA at the same time point.

that contained the 884-bp fragment of the promoter region of the CCL5 gene and multiple binding sites for NF-κB. The cells were transfected with these plasmids, as described previously [11, 12], and incubated for 24 h. We then added poly I:C and cytokines, collected the cells 24 h later and stored them at –80°C until measuring the luciferase activity with the Dual-Luciferase Assay System (Promega). The firefly-luciferase activity of the reporter plasmid was normalized to Renilla-luciferase activity, expressed as fold induction, and compared with a control.

Knock Down of Gene Expression Using Short Interfering RNA
Pre-designed short interfering RNAs (siRNAs) for signal transducer and activator of transcription 1 (STAT-1) and negative control of siRNA (scrambled siRNA) were purchased from Ambion (Tokyo, Japan). The cells were transfected with 50 nM of each siRNA with 5 μl Lipofectamine 2000 (Promega), as described previously [11–13]. After 48 h, the cells were stimulated with poly I:C and cytokines. Twenty-four hours after stimulation, we harvested the cells and collected the supernatants.

Assay of the Stability of CCL5 mRNA
We treated the cells for 8 h with dsRNA alone or with dsRNA in combination with either TNF-α or IFN-γ. Afterwards, we either harvested the cells at time 0 (representing the control condition) or further treated them with the transcriptional inhibitor actinomycin D (Sigma) for 4 or 8 h and then harvested the cells. We used real-time PCR to analyze the levels of CCL5 mRNA, as described above, and expressed it as percent of the level at time 0.

Western Blotting
Western blotting was performed to investigate the activation of STAT-1, as described previously [11, 14]. We then subjected whole-cell extracts to 10% Tris-glycine gradient gel electrophoresis (Novex, San Diego, Calif., USA) and transferred the extract to a nitrocellulose membrane (Schleicher & Schuell, Dassel, Germany). The membranes were blocked with 5% non-fat milk powder in TBST (50 mM Tris, 0.15 M NaCl and 0.05% Tween 20), incubated with 1 μg/ml rabbit anti-STAT-1 antibody (Ab) or anti-phospho-STAT-1 (Santa Cruz Biotechnology, Santa Cruz, Calif., USA) in TBST for 3 h, washed with TBST and then incubated with anti-rabbit Ig Ab (Amersham Biosciences, Tokyo, Japan) for 1 h. After extensive washing with TBST, we added a chemiluminescent substrate (ECL Western blot detection system, Amersham Biosciences) and subjected the membrane to autoradiography. Densitometry was employed to analyze the intensity of the bands, and the ratio was calculated by dividing the intensity of phosphorylated STAT-1 by the intensity of STAT-1.

Statistical Analysis
Data were expressed as means ± SEM. Statistical differences were determined by analysis of variance with Fisher's protected least significant difference test. Data were analyzed with StatView IV software (Abacus Concepts, Berkeley, Calif., USA.

Results

Synergistic or Additive Effects of TNF-α or IFN-γ on CCL5 Expression with dsRNA
The expression of CCL5 mRNA or CCL5 protein was up-regulated after stimulation with dsRNA. TNF-α modestly stimulated CCL5 expression, but TNF-α combined with dsRNA additively up-regulated CCL5 expression. Maximum expression was observed 12–24 h after stimulation (fig. 1). Very low levels of CCL5 mRNA or CCL5 protein were detected in cells stimulated by IFN-γ alone. However, IFN-γ significantly up-regulated dsRNA-induced CCL5 expression. Maximum expression occurred 8–24 h after stimulation (fig. 2).

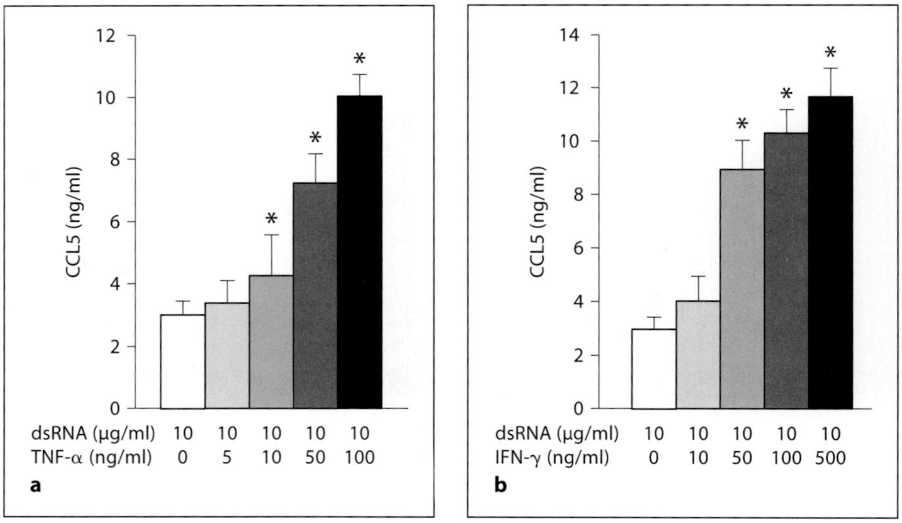

Fig. 3. Effect of different doses of TNF-α or IFN-γ on CCL5 protein expression induced by dsRNA. BEAS-2B cells were incubated with synthetic dsRNA poly I:C (10 μg/ml) and the indicated doses of TNF-α (**a**) or IFN-γ (**b**) for 24 h and analyzed by ELISA. Means ± SEM of three independent experiments. * $p < 0.05$ vs. cells stimulated with dsRNA only.

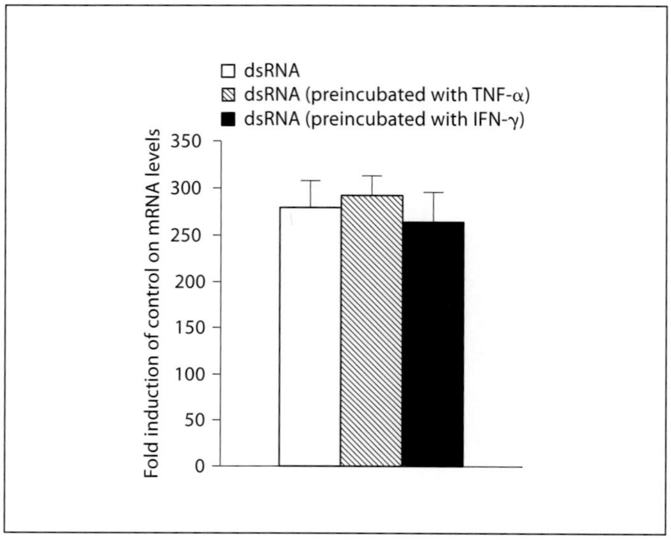

Fig. 4. Effect of preincubation with TNF-α or IFN-γ on CCL5 mRNA expression induced by dsRNA. BEAS-2B cells were preincubated with or without TNF-α (10 ng/ml) or IFN-γ (50 ng/ml) for 24 h and then incubated with synthetic dsRNA poly I:C (10 μg/ml) after medium exchange prior to real-time PCR. Means ± SEM of three independent experiments.

Dose-Dependent Relationship of TNF-α or IFN-γ on dsRNA-Induced CCL5 Expression

The expression of CCL5 protein was up-regulated after stimulation with TNF-α (fig. 3a) or IFN-γ (fig. 3b) in a dose-dependent manner in the presence of dsRNA poly I:C (10 μg/ml) 24 h after stimulation.

Effects of Preincubation with TNF-α or IFN-γ on the Expression of CCL5 mRNA

To analyze priming effects of TNF-α or IFN-γ, BEAS-2B cells were treated with TNF-α or IFN-γ for 24 h and then the medium was changed. Cells were stimulated with dsRNA poly I:C (10 μg/ml), collected 24 h after stimulation and then subjected to real-time PCR. However, preincubation with TNF-α or IFN-γ did not affect the expression of CCL5 mRNA in the presence of dsRNA (fig. 4).

TNF-α Activates the Promoter Region of CCL5, but IFN-γ Does Not Activate It

TNF-α alone or dsRNA alone stimulated the activity of the CCL5 promoter region (which contains binding sites for NF-κB). The combination of TNF-α and dsRNA additively stimulated the CCL5 promoter region (fig. 5a). These data were compatible with the data of CCL5 mRNA and CCL5 protein. Similar data were observed in the NF-κB reporter, indicating that the additive effect of TNF-α and dsRNA on CCL5 expression may depend on their cooperative activation of NF-κB (fig. 5b). On the other

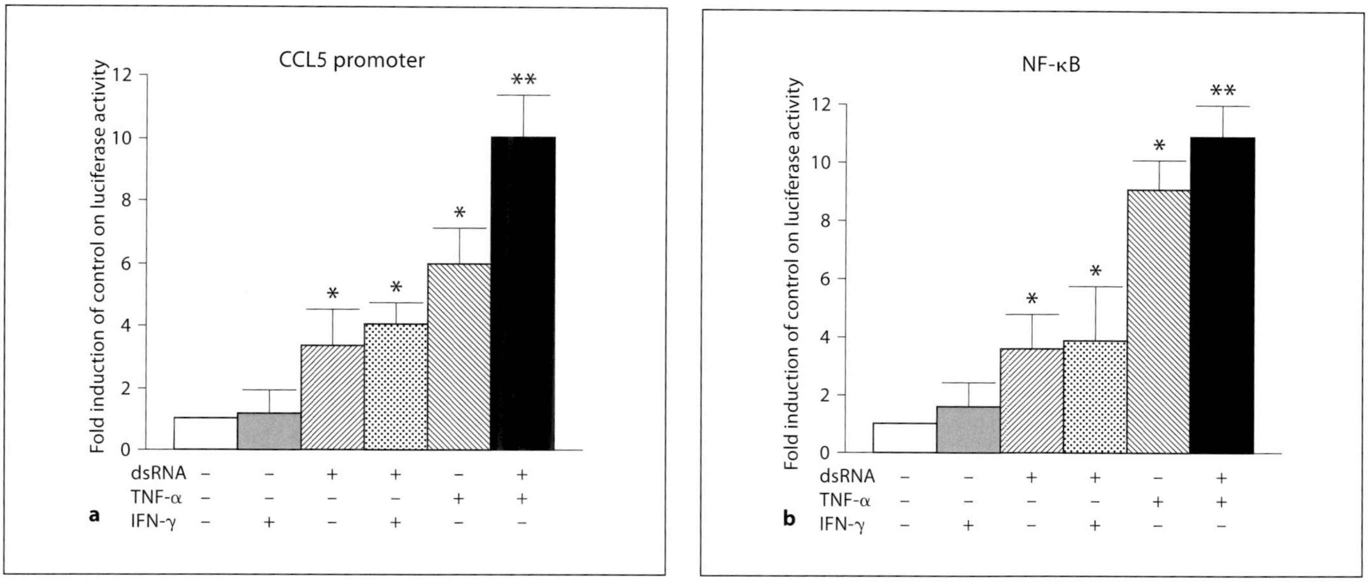

Fig. 5. Effect of TNF-α (10 ng/ml), IFN-γ (50 ng/ml) and dsRNA poly I:C (10 μg/ml) on CCL5 promoter activity (**a**) and the NF-κB reporter (**b**). BEAS-2B cells were transfected with the CCL5/RANTES promoter-luciferase reporter plasmids and control vector pRL-TK. Forty-eight hours later, cells were incubated for 24 h either with or without the indicated cytokines or dsRNA. The relative luciferase activity was calculated as fold induction, compared with the control value. Means ± SEM of three independent experiments. * $p < 0.05$ vs. non-stimulated control cells; ** $p < 0.05$ vs. cells stimulated with dsRNA.

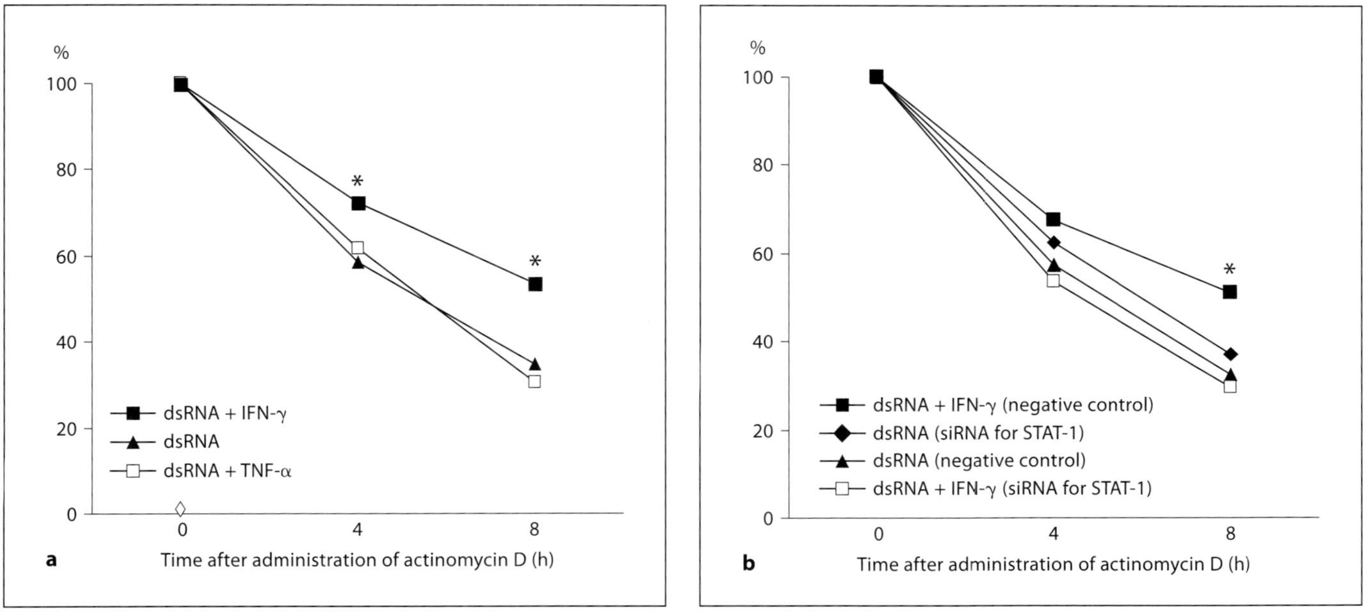

Fig. 6. Stability of CCL5 mRNA after stimulation with dsRNA poly I:C (10 μg/ml) and/or IFN-γ (50 ng/ml) or TNF-α (10ng/ml) in BEAS-2B cells (**a**) or in cells transfected with siRNA for STAT-1 or a negative control (**b**). Cells were treated for 8 h and then either harvested at time 0 (as a control) or further treated with actinomycin D for 4 or 8 h prior to real-time PCR. Means ± SEM of three independent experiments. * $p < 0.05$ vs. cells treated with dsRNA.

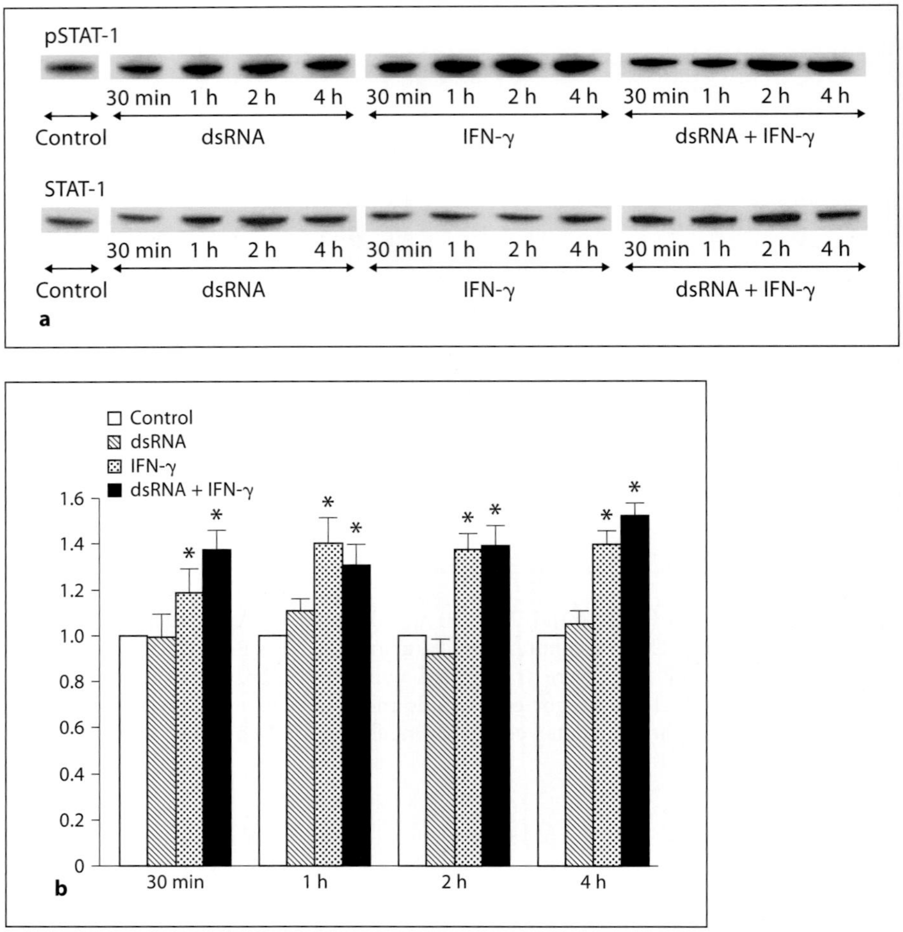

Fig. 7. Result of the Western blot for the expression of STAT-1 protein (STAT-1) or phosphorylated STAT-1 (pSTAT-1). BEAS-2B cells were stimulated either with or without dsRNA poly I:C (10 μg/ml), IFN-γ (50 ng/ml) or dsRNA plus IFN-γ for 30 min to 4 h. **a** Whole-cell extracts were collected and then subjected to Western blotting. **b** The intensity of each band was analyzed by densitometry and the pSTAT-1/STAT-1 ratio was calculated. Means ± SEM of three independent experiments. * $p < 0.05$ vs. non-treated cells.

hand, IFN-γ did not stimulate the activity of the CCL5 promoter region. IFN-γ combined with dsRNA did not increase the activation of the CCL5 promoter region (fig. 5a). These results indicate that IFN-γ may regulate the post-transcription of the CCL5 gene.

IFN-γ Stabilizes CCL5 mRNA Expression Induced by dsRNA

After stimulation with dsRNA, the level of CCL5 mRNA decreased with actinomycin D treatment (fig. 6a). After stimulation with the combination of dsRNA and IFN-γ, the level of CCL5 mRNA was higher than its level after dsRNA stimulation alone. This effect did not occur in cells stimulated with the combination of dsRNA and TNF-α (fig. 6a) or in cells transfected with siRNA for STAT-1 and then stimulated with the combination of dsRNA and IFN-γ (fig. 6b). These data indicate that IFN-γ may stabilize dsRNA-induced CCL5 mRNA expression through activation of STAT-1.

Phosphorylation of STAT-1 by IFN-γ

IFN-γ phosphorylated STAT-1 in BEAS-2 cells from 30 min to 2 h (fig. 7). Stimulation with dsRNA did not phosphorylate STAT-1 and, therefore, did not change the level of phosphorylated STAT-1. These results indicate that activation of STAT-1 may depend on IFN-γ stimulation alone.

Effect of STAT-1 Inhibition on the Expression of CCL5 mRNA and CCL5 Protein

BEAS-2B cells transfected with siRNA for STAT-1 had significantly down-regulated the level of STAT-1 mRNA (data not shown). The negative control of siRNA did not interfere with the expression of STAT-1 mRNA. The cooperative activation of the combination of IFN-γ and dsRNA on the expression of CCL5 mRNA (fig. 8a) or CCL5 protein (fig. 8b) in BEAS-2B cells was down-regulated in the cells transfected with siRNA for STAT-1. These data indicate that STAT-1 may be important in the regulation of CCL5 expression by IFN-γ in airway epithelial cells.

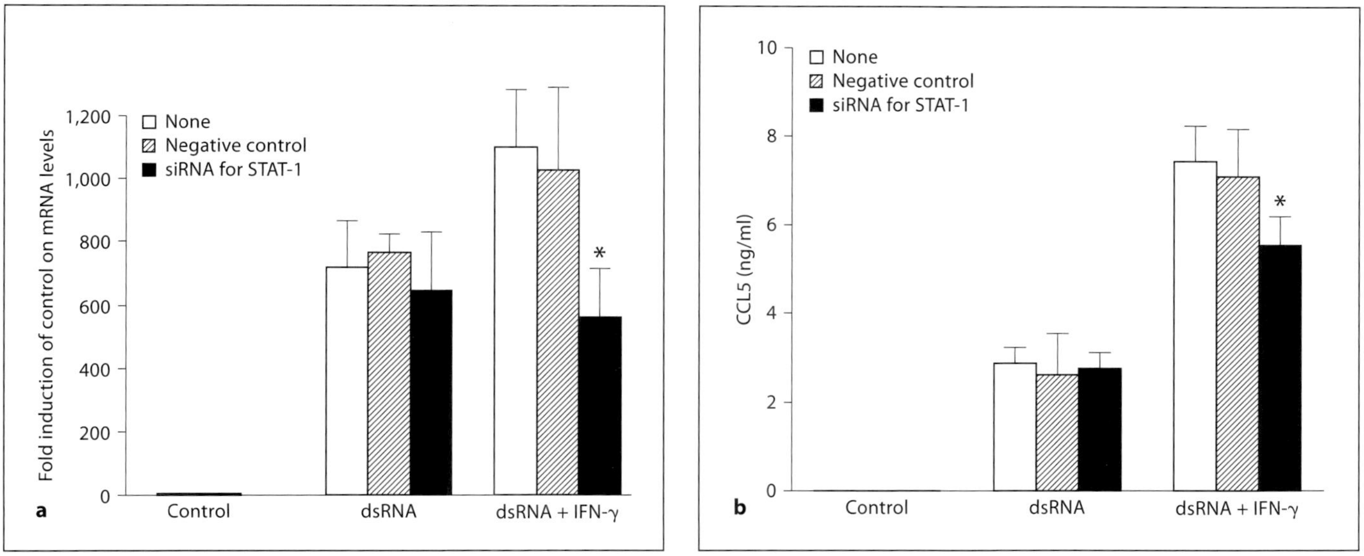

Fig. 8. Effect of siRNA for STAT-1 or a negative control on CCL5 mRNA expression (**a**) and CCL5 protein expression (**b**). BEAS-2B cells were transfected with siRNA for STAT-1 or a negative control. Non-transfected cells and transfected cells were treated with dsRNA poly I:C (10 μg/ml) or dsRNA (10 μg/ml) plus IFN-γ (50 ng/ml) for 8 h for PCR or for 24 h for ELISA. Means ± SEM of three independent experiments. * $p < 0.05$ vs. non-transfected cells.

Discussion

We demonstrate that the inflammatory cytokines TNF-α and IFN-γ, in cooperation with a ligand of TLR3 dsRNA, up-regulate the expression of the chemokine CCL5/RANTES in airway epithelial cells. In this mechanism, TNF-α may additively activate NF-κB, which is a key transcription factor regulating the CCL5 promoter region. IFN-γ may not directly regulate the transcription of CCL5, but it stabilizes CCL5 dsRNA-induced mRNA expression through activation of STAT-1.

Several reports indicate the priming effects of TNF-α or IFN-γ on TLR signaling. These cytokines up-regulate the expression of receptors for dsRNA, such as TLR3, dsRNA-dependent protein kinase (PKR), melanoma differentiation-associated gene 5 (MDA-5) and retinoic acid-inducible gene 1 (RIG-1) [15, 16]. We have also confirmed that TNF-α up-regulated TLR3 mRNA expression in airway epithelial cells [unpubl. data]. We then hypothesized that up-regulation of TLR3 expression by cytokines may contribute to the hyperresponsiveness to dsRNA and subsequent cooperative activation of CCL5 expression. In this study, we examined the effects of pretreatment with TNF-α or IFN-γ on CCL5 expression in epithelial cells stimulated with dsRNA. However, we could not detect any priming effects. Moreover, the effects of these cytokines under dsRNA stimulation were different among the various target genes. For example, IFN-γ did not stimulate CXCL8/IL-8 expression induced by dsRNA [unpubl. data]. Taken together, up-regulation of TLR3 mRNA expression may not contribute to the cooperative up-regulation of CCL5 with dsRNA and TNF-α/IFN-γ in our study.

NF-κB reportedly activates the transcription of CCL5 in response to TNF-α, viral infection and dsRNA [11, 17, 18]. Our result showing an additive activation of NF-κB by the combination of TNF-α and dsRNA and the subsequent stimulation of CCL5 transcription may be concordant with previous reports. Other transcription factors, such as AP-1, may regulate CCL5 transcription in response to TNF-α and/or dsRNA. However, AP-1 did not activate CCL5 expression in our previous studies [11, 12]. Some reports suggest constitutive activation of NF-κB in the airway epithelium of asthmatics [19]. Therefore, the excessive response to a virus and overexpression of CCL5 may easily occur in asthma exacerbation induced by viral infection.

IFN-γ activates transcription factors such as STAT-1 and IRF-1. STAT-1 homodimers bind to the γ-activated sequence element of DNA in the promoter region of a target gene. IRF-1 expression can be directly activated by IFN-γ or up-regulated by IFN-γ through STAT-1. Activated IRF-1 binds the IFN-stimulated response element of DNA in the promoter region of the target gene. Several reports indicate that STAT-1 or IRF-1 binds to the promoter region of CCL5 and stimulates its activity [20–22]. In our study, however, IFN-γ did not stimulate the CCL5 promoter either with or without dsRNA stimulation. Further studies are needed to clarify this discrepancy. One reason may be related to the differences among the various cell types.

We next focused on the post-transcriptional regulation of CCL5 by IFN-γ. Stellato et al. [3] first reported CCL5 expression in airway epithelial cells and suggested that IFN-γ in combination with TNF-α may stabilize CCL5 mRNA. IFN-γ also stabilizes other genes [23] and dsRNA-induced expression of CCL5 mRNA. To investigate this mechanism, we further observed STAT-1, which transduces the initial signal of IFN-γ [24]. IFN-γ phosphorylated STAT-1 in BEAS-2B cells and the effect of IFN-γ was not evident in the cells in which siRNA had down-regulated STAT-1 expression. Further studies are required to clarify how STAT-1 translates the IFN-γ signal and how it stabilizes CCL5 mRNA induced by dsRNA. However, we hypothesize that STAT-1 may interact with RNA-binding protein and may regulate the post-transcriptional modulation of CCL5 RNA. STAT-3 is associated with Sam68 (an RNA-binding protein) in response to leptin [25]. The up-regulation of STAT-1 in the airway epithelium of asthmatics indicates the possible expression of CCL5 during viral infection in asthma [26].

Our results show the cross-talk between inflammatory cytokines and TLR3 in airway epithelial cells. Epithelial-derived CCL5 may play an important role in host defense against viral infections. However, CCL5 overexpression may contribute to the pathogenesis of airway inflammation, including asthma exacerbation. Further investigation of these mechanisms may contribute to the understanding of airway diseases.

Acknowledgments

The authors would like to thank Dr. Tomas J. Schall for providing CCL5/RANTES promoter plasmid and Drs. Fumio Kokubu, Tsutomu Hirano and Takeshi Kasama for their excellent assistance and helpful discussions. This work was supported by the Environmental Restoration and Conservation Agency and GlaxoSmithKline.

Disclosure Statement

The authors declare that no financial or other conflict of interest exists in relation to the content of this article.

References

1 Dougherty R, Fahy J: Acute exacerbations of asthma: epidemiology, biology and the exacerbation-prone phenotype. Clin Exp Allergy 2009;39:193–202.

2 Gern J: Viral respiratory infection and the link to asthma. Pediatr Infect Dis J 2008; 27(suppl 10):S97-S103.

3 Stellato C, Beck L, Gorgone G, Proud D, Schall T, Ono S, Lichtenstein L, Schleimer R: Expression of the chemokine RANTES by a human bronchial epithelial cell line. Modulation by cytokines and glucocorticoids. J Immunol 1995;155:410–418.

4 Puthothu B, Bierbaum S, Kopp M, Forster J, Heinze J, Weckmann M, Krueger M, Heinzmann A: Association of TNF-alpha with severe respiratory syncytial virus infection and bronchial asthma. Pediatr Allergy Immunol 2009;20:157–163.

5 van Schaik S, Tristram D, Nagpal I, Hintz K, Welliver R 2nd, Welliver R: Increased production of IFN-gamma and cysteinyl leukotrienes in virus-induced wheezing. J Allergy Clin Immunol 1999;103:630–636.

6 Matsukura S, Kokubu F, Noda H, Tokunaga H, Adachi M: Expression of IL-6, IL-8, and RANTES on human bronchial epithelial cells, NCI-H292, induced by influenza virus A. J Allergy Clin Immunol 1996;98:1080–1087.

7 Matsukura S, Kokubu F, Kubo H, Tomita T, Tokunaga H, Kadokura M, Yamamoto T, Kuroiwa Y, Ohno T, Suzaki H, Adachi M: Expression of RANTES by normal airway epithelial cells after influenza virus A infection. Am J Respir Cell Mol Biol 1998;18:255–264.

8 Veckman V, Osterlund P, Fagerlund R, Melén K, Matikainen S, Julkunen I: TNF-alpha and IFN-alpha enhance influenza-A-virus-induced chemokine gene expression in human A549 lung epithelial cells. Virology 2006;345:96–104.

9 Konno S, Grindle K, Lee W, Schroth M, Mosser A, Brockman-Schneider R, Busse W, Gern J: Interferon-gamma enhances rhinovirus-induced RANTES secretion by airway epithelial cells. Am J Respir Cell Mol Biol 2002;26:594–601.

10 Olszewska-Pazdrak B, Casola A, Saito T, Alam R, Crowe S, Mei F, Ogra P, Garofalo R: Cell-specific expression of RANTES, MCP-1, and MIP-1α by lower airway epithelial cells and eosinophils infected with respiratory syncytial virus. J Virol 1998;72:4756–4764.

11 Ieki K, Matsukura S, Kokubu F, Kimura T, Kuga H, Kawaguchi M, Odaka M, Suzuki S, Watanabe S, Takeuchi H, Schleimer R, Adachi M: Double-stranded RNA activates RANTES gene transcription through co-operation of nuclear factor-kappa B and interferon regulatory factors in human airway epithelial cells. Clin Exp Allergy 2004;34: 745–752.

12 Matsukura S, Kokubu F, Kurokawa M, Kawaguchi M, Ieki K, Kuga H, Odaka M, Suzuki S, Watanabe S, Takeuchi H, Kasama T, Adachi M: Synthetic double-stranded RNA induces multiple genes related to inflammation through Toll-like receptor 3 depending on NF-kappa B and/or IRF-3 in airway epithelial cells. Clin Exp Allergy 2006;36:1049–1062.

13 Matsukura S, Kokubu F, Kurokawa M, Kawaguchi M, Ieki K, Kuga H, Odaka M, Suzuki S, Watanabe S, Homma T, Takeuchi H, Nohtomi K, Adachi M: Role of RIG-I, MDA-5, and PKR on the expression of inflammatory chemokines induced by synthetic dsRNA in airway epithelial cells. Int Arch Allergy Immunol 2007;143(suppl 1):80–83.
14 Matsukura S, Stellato C, Georas SN, Casolaro V, Plitt JR, Miura K, Kurosawa S, Schindler U, Schleimer RP: Interleukin-13 upregulates eotaxin expression in airway epithelial cells by a STAT6-dependent mechanism. Am J Respir Cell Mol Biol 2001;24: 755–761.
15 Kawai T, Akira S: Toll-like receptor and RIG-I-like receptor signaling. Ann NY Acad Sci 2008;1143:1–20.
16 Schroder K, Hertzog P, Ravasi T, Hume D: Interferon-gamma: an overview of signals, mechanisms and functions. J Leukoc Biol 2004;75:163–189.
17 Genin P, Algarte M, Roof P, Lin R, Hiscott J: Regulation of RANTES chemokine gene expression requires cooperativity between NF-κB and IFN-regulatory factor transcription factors. J Immunol 2000;164:5352–5361.
18 Casola A, Garofalo R, Haeberle H, Elliott T, Lin R, Jamaluddin M, Brasier A: Multiple cis regulatory elements control RANTES promoter activity in alveolar epithelial cells infected with respiratory syncytial virus. J Virol 2001;75:6428–6439.
19 Hart L, Krishnan V, Adcock I, Barnes P, Chung K: Activation and localization of transcription factor, nuclear factor-κB, in asthma. Am J Respir Crit Care Med 1998; 158:1585–1592.
20 Liu J, Guan X, Ma X: Interferon regulatory factor 1 is an essential and direct transcriptional activator for interferon γ-induced RANTES/CCl5 expression in macrophages. J Biol Chem 2005;280:24347–24355.
21 Lee A, Hong J, Seo Y: Tumour necrosis factor-alpha and interferon-gamma synergistically activate the RANTES promoter through nuclear factor kappa B and interferon regulatory factor 1 (IRF-1) transcription factors. Biochem J 2000;350:131–138.
22 Ohmori Y, Schreiber R, Hamilton T: Synergy between interferon-gamma and tumor necrosis factor-alpha in transcriptional activation is mediated by cooperation between signal transducer and activator of transcription 1 and nuclear factor kappa B. J Biol Chem 1997;272:14899–14907.
23 Yip-Schneider M, Horie M, Broxmeyer H: Transcriptional induction of pim-1 protein kinase gene expression by interferon gamma and posttranscriptional effects on costimulation with steel factor. Blood 1995;85:3494–3502.
24 Darnell J: STATs and gene regulation. Science 1997;277:1630–1635.
25 Sánchez-Margalet V, Martín-Romero C, Santos-Alvarez J, Goberna R, Najib S, Gonzalez-Yanes C: Role of leptin as an immunomodulator of blood mononuclear cells: mechanisms of action. Clin Exp Immunol 2003;133:11–19.
26 Sampath D, Castro M, Look D, Holtzman M: Constitutive activation of an epithelial signal transducer and activator of transcription (STAT) pathway in asthma. J Clin Invest 1999;103:1353–1361.

Original Paper

International Archives of Allergy and Immunology

Int Arch Allergy Immunol 2010;152(suppl 1):18–21
DOI: 10.1159/000312121

Published online: June 4, 2010

Selective Down-Regulation of Th2 Cytokines by C-Terminal Binding Protein 2 in Human T Cells

Fujiko Kitamura[a] Noriko Kitamura[c] Akio Mori[c] Hideki Tatsumi[d] Soichi Nemoto[d] Hiroyuki Miyoshi[e] Shoichiro Miyatake[b] Takachika Hiroi[a] Osamu Kaminuma[a]

[a]Department of Allergy and Immunology, and [b]Cytokine Project, Tokyo Metropolitan Institute of Medical Science, Tokyo, [c]Clinical Research Center for Allergy and Rheumatology, and [d]Department of Obstetrics and Gynecology, National Hospital Organization, Sagamihara National Hospital, Sagamihara, and [e]Subteam for Manipulation of Cell Fate, BioResource Center, RIKEN, Tsukuba Institute, Tsukuba, Japan

Key Words

CtBP · FOG · GATA-3 · Human T cells · Th1/Th2

Abstract

Background: Among several C-terminal binding proteins (CtBPs), friend of GATA (FOG) has been implicated in the down-regulation of GATA-3-mediated Th2 cell differentiation. Here we investigated the role of CtBP2 in Th1 and Th2 cytokine expression in human T cells. ***Methods:*** CtBP2 was introduced into human peripheral CD4+ T cells by a lentiviral transduction system. Subsequently, the expression of Th1 and Th2 cytokine mRNA was determined by quantitative real-time RT-PCR. ***Results:*** CtBP2 significantly suppressed stimulation-induced expression of IL-4, IL-5 and IL-13 in human T cells. However, IFN-γ expression was not affected by the introduction of CtBP2. ***Conclusion:*** CtBP2 selectively down-regulates Th2 cytokines, therefore it is a potential target for the treatment of allergic diseases.

Introduction

CD4+ T cells are classified into at least four distinct subsets, Th1, Th2, Th17 and regulatory T cells [1]. Among them, Th2 cells preferentially secrete IL-4, IL-5 and IL-13, and are counteractive to Th1 cells. As Th2 cytokines are essential for IgE synthesis, eosinophil activation and mucus hypersecretion, Th2 cells are crucially involved in allergic diseases [1].

Like other CD4+ T cell subsets, the development of Th2 cells is strictly regulated by their specific transcription factor, GATA-3 [1]. GATA-3 enhances the expression of several Th2 cytokines through the GATA sites present in their *cis*-regulatory elements [2]. In addition, this transcription factor induces an accessible chromatin configuration at the IL-4 loci which harbor IL-4, IL-13 and IL-5 [3]. Therefore, down-regulation of GATA-3 activity is promising to treat allergic diseases.

It has been reported that GATA-3-dependent development of Th2 cells was suppressed by a multitype zinc finger protein, friend of GATA (FOG). Thus, retroviral introduction of FOG into murine naive T cells repressed the development of Th2 cells [4, 5]. Furthermore, the pro-

KARGER

Fax +41 61 306 12 34
E-Mail karger@karger.ch
www.karger.com

© 2010 S. Karger AG, Basel
1018–2438/10/1525–0018$26.00/0

Accessible online at:
www.karger.com/iaa

Correspondence to: Dr. Osamu Kaminuma, Department of Allergy and Immunology
Tokyo Metropolitan Institute of Medical Science
2-1-6 Kamikitazawa, Setagaya-ku, Tokyo 156-8506 (Japan)
Tel. +81 3 5316 3126, ext. 2670, Fax +81 3 5316 3153
E-Mail kaminuma-os@igakuken.or.jp

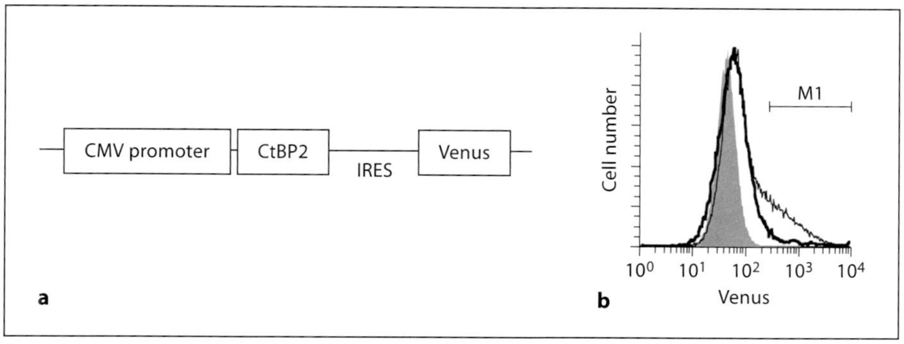

Fig. 1. Introduction of CtBP2 into human CD4+ T cells. **a** A serial expression cassette containing CMV promoter-driven CtBP2-IRES-Venus (CtBP2) was introduced into peripheral-blood naïve CD4+ T cells by a lentivirus infection system during stimulation culture. **b** Then the resulting Venus-positive population (M1) in CtBP2 (thick line) and empty IRES-Venus (vector: thin line) was purified. The gray area indicates untransfected background.

moter activities of IL-4 and IL-5 were down-regulated by FOG in a human T-cell line (Jurkat [5]). Even though the mechanisms underlying FOG-mediated down-regulation of GATA-3 activity have not been elucidated, FOG associates with a transcriptional co-repressor, C-terminal binding protein (CtBP) [6, 7].

CtBP family members, originally discovered as a cellular protein that interacted with the C-terminus of adenovirus E1A proteins [8], are highly conserved in invertebrates and vertebrates [9]. Genetic studies indicate that the CtBP genes play pivotal roles in animal development [10]. CtBP proteins are broadly expressed and have been implicated in multiple intracellular signaling and transcriptional control pathways, as well as cell survival and tumorigenesis [9, 11]. However, the functional role of CtBPs in immune responses has not been elucidated in detail.

The various DNA-binding repressors recruit CtBPs through PxDLS-like motifs [8]. Among CtBP family members, CtBP2 has been shown to interact with FOG through its PIDLS sequence [6, 7]. In addition, FOG-mediated suppression of GATA activity was diminished by mutation in this motif [12], suggesting that CtBP2 plays a role in Th1/Th2 development by affecting FOG/GATA-3-mediated regulatory pathway(s) in Th2 cytokine genes.

In order to elucidate the functional role of CtBP2 in T-cell cytokine synthesis, we here investigated the contribution of CtBP2 to Th1 and Th2 cytokine expression in human peripheral CD4+ T cells, employing a lentiviral transduction system and quantitative real-time RT-PCR.

Methods

Plasmid Constructs and Lentivirus Preparation

The PCR fragment of cDNA encoding full-length human CtBP2 (amino acids 1–446) was subcloned in frame into an appropriate site in the CMV promoter-driven lentivirus expression vector combined with an internal ribosomal entry site (IRES) followed by the coding sequence of a luminescent protein, Venus, at the C-terminal end (fig. 1a) [13, 14]. The correct sequence of the construct was verified by sequencing. Lentiviruses pseudotyped with vesicular stomatitis virus G glycoprotein were prepared as described previously [15].

Cells, Lentivirus Infection and Transfection

With approval by the Ethics Committee of the Tokyo Metropolitan Institute of Medical Science and the Sagamihara National Hospital, CD4+CD45RO− naïve T cells were prepared from the peripheral blood of healthy volunteers purified by a combination of negative and positive selection using CD45RO and CD4 microbeads, respectively, with a magnetic cell-sorting system (Miltenyi Biotec, Bergisch Gladbach, Germany). The purity of resulting cells was >99% as determined by flow cytometry. Naïve T cells were cultured in AIM-V medium (Invitrogen) in the presence of 0.01 μg/ml anti-CD3 antibody (Ab) OKT3 (Ortho Biotech Products, Bridgewater, N.J., USA), 1 μg/ml anti-CD28 Ab (BD Bioscience, San Jose, Calif., USA) and 10 U/ml recombinant IL-2 (Shionogi, Osaka, Japan). No additional Th1/Th2 cytokine or its Ab was added, since human peripheral naïve T cells produce both Th1 and Th2 cytokines after stimulation culture under neutral conditions [15]. For protein overexpression, cells were infected with viral stock solutions at a multiplicity of infection of 50–200 at 24 h after the start of culture. After 7–10 days of stimulation, lentivirus infection-positive cells were purified with a FACSArea cell-sorting system (BD Bioscience).

Messenger RNA Expression

Total RNA was extracted from T cells stimulated with 5 nM phorbol 12-myristate 13-acetate (PMA) and 1 μM ionomycin for 6 h at 37°C. After reverse transcription using oligo(dT)12–18 primer and ReverTra ACE (Toyobo, Osaka, Japan), quantitative real-time RT-PCR for IL-4, IL-5, IL-13 and IFN-γ was performed using Assay-on-Demand™ Gene Expression Products (TaqMan® MGB probes) with an ABI Prism 7900 sequence detection system (Applied Biosystems, Foster City, Calif., USA).

Statistical Analysis

Results are expressed as arithmetic means ± SEM. Statistical analysis was performed by Student's t test. $p < 0.05$ was considered to indicate statistical significance.

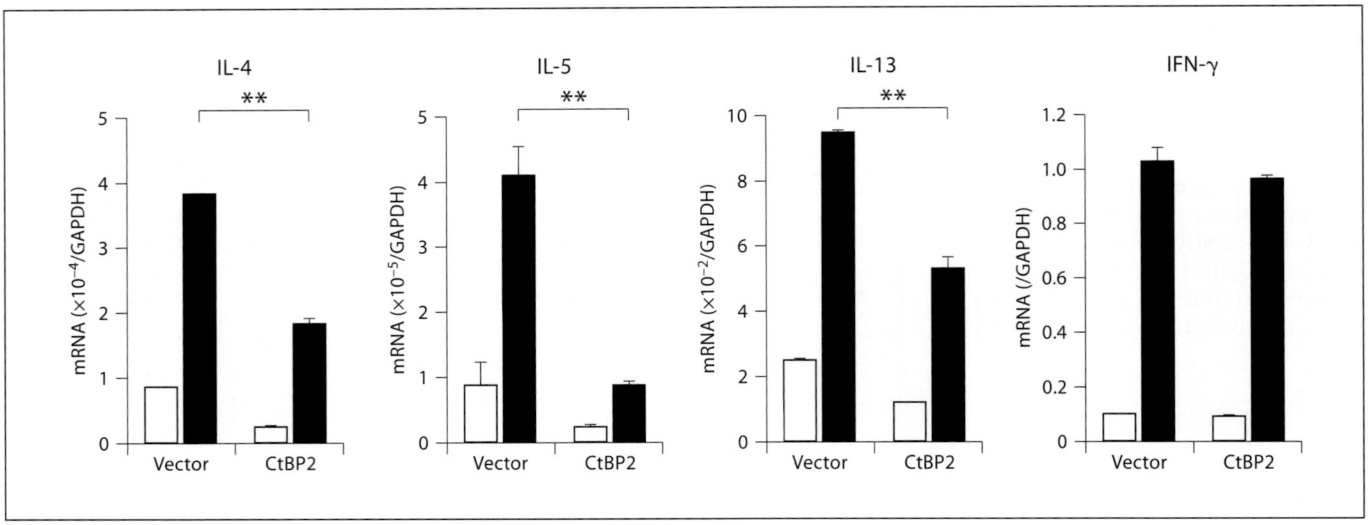

Fig. 2. The purified Venus-positive cells were left unstimulated (□) or stimulated with 5 nM PMA plus 1 μM ionomycin (■) for 6 h, and the expression of IL-4, IL-5, IL-13 and IFN-γ mRNA was measured by means of quantitative real-time RT-PCR. Means ± SEM of mRNA abundance normalized to GAPDH expression (n = 4). ** $p < 0.01$.

Results and Discussion

The effect of CtBP2 on Th1 and Th2 expression was elucidated at the mRNA level. CtBP2 conjunct with Venus through IRES was introduced into peripheral-blood CD4+ T cells by a lentivirus infection system; then the transduction-positive population (M1 in fig. 1b) was purified by cell sorting. On stimulation with phorbol ester plus Ca^{2}+ ionophore, the expression of IL-4, IL-5, IL-13 and IFN-γ was significantly augmented in these cells (fig. 2). The stimulation-induced expression of all Th2 cytokines examined was clearly suppressed by the introduction of CtBP2. Especially IL-5 expression was most severely diminished. These findings are consistent with previous reports demonstrating that GATA-3-mediated Th2 development was suppressed by FOG [4, 5], which utilizes CtBPs to exhibit its transcription repressor activity [12], and that IL-5 expression was especially dependent on GATA-3 [16].

On the other hand, CtBP2 failed to affect the expression of IFN-γ (fig. 2). It seems a little strange that only Th2 cytokines were affected by CtBP2, since Th1 and Th2 cytokines have been recognized to counteract each other [1]. However, this Th1/Th2 paradigm, chiefly established by murine studies, does not always apply for human T-cell differentiation. It may be caused, at least in part, by genetic and epigenetic regulation of Th1/Th2 cytokine gene loci as well as differential expression of Th1- and Th2-type transcription factors specifically in human T cells [17–19]. Although Th2 cytokines are significantly up-regulated in CD4+ T cells of patients with allergic asthma, IFN-γ expression was unchanged in those cells [15]. Interestingly, Kurata et al. [5] reported that the promoter activity not only of IL-4 and IL-5 but also of IFN-γ in Jurkat T cells was suppressed by overexpression of FOG. Further investigations will be required, therefore, in order to elucidate additional details on the functional contribution of the CtBP2/FOG/GATA-3-related transcription pathway to IFN-γ synthesis in human CD4+ T cells.

In conclusion, CtBP2 may be of benefit in the treatment of allergic diseases including bronchial asthma, due to its specific contribution to the down-regulation of Th2 cytokine synthesis in human T cells.

Acknowledgments

We thank Dr. A. Miyawaki for providing Venus. This work was supported in part by the Japan Allergy Foundation (to O.K.) and the Nisshin Seifun Foundation (to O.K.).

Disclosure Statement

The authors declare that no financial or other conflict of interest exists in relation to the content of this article.

References

1 Zhu J, Paul WE: CD4 T cells: fates, functions, and faults. Blood 2008;112:1557–1569.

2 Zheng DH, Flavell RA: The transcription factor GATA-3 is necessary and sufficient for Th2 cytokine gene expression in CD4 T cells. Cell 1997;89:587–596.

3 Lee GR, Fields PE, Flavell RA: Regulation of IL-4 gene expression by distal regulatory elements and GATA-3 at the chromatin level. Immunity 2001;14:447–459.

4 Zhou M, Ouyang W, Gong Q, Katz SG, White JM, Orkin SH, Murphy KM: Friend of GATA-1 represses GATA-3-dependent activity in CD4+ T cells. J Exp Med 2001;194:1461–1471.

5 Kurata H, Lee HJ, McClanahan T, Coffman RL, O'Garra A, Arai N: Friend of GATA is expressed in naive Th cells and functions as a repressor of GATA-3-mediated Th2 cell development. J Immunol 2002;168:4538–4545.

6 Turner J, Crossley M: Cloning and characterization of mCtBP2, a co-repressor that associates with basic Krüppel-like factor and other mammalian transcriptional regulators. EMBO J 1998;17:5129–5140.

7 Holmes M, Turner J, Fox A, Chisholm O, Crossley M, Chong B: hFOG2, a novel zinc finger protein, binds the co-repressor mCtBP2 and modulates GATA-mediated activation. J Biol Chem 1999;274:23491–23498.

8 Schaeper U, Boyd JM, Verma S, Uhlmann E, Subramanian T, Chinnadurai G: Molecular cloning and characterization of a cellular phosphoprotein that interacts with a conserved C-terminal domain of adenovirus E1A involved in negative modulation of oncogenic transformation. Proc Natl Acad Sci USA 1995;92:10467–10471.

9 Chinnadurai G: CtBP, an unconventional transcriptional corepressor in development and oncogenesis. Mol Cell 2002;9:213–224.

10 Hildebrand JD, Soriano P: Overlapping and unique roles for C-terminal binding protein 1 (CtBP1) and CtBP2 during mouse development. Mol Cell Biol 2002;22:5296–5307.

11 Bergman LM, Blaydes JP: C-terminal binding proteins: emerging roles in cell survival and tumorigenesis. Apoptosis 2006;11:879–888.

12 Fox AH, Liew C, Holmes M, Kowalski K, Mackay J, Crossley M: Transcriptional cofactors of the FOG family interact with GATA proteins by means of multiple zinc fingers. EMBO J 1999;18:2812–2822.

13 Miyoshi H, Blomer U, Takahashi M, Gage FH, Verma IM: Development of a self-inactivating lentivirus vector. J Virol 1998;72:8150–8157.

14 Nagai T, Ibata K, Park ES, Kubota M, Mikoshiba K, Miyawaki A: A variant of yellow fluorescent protein with fast and efficient maturation for cell-biological applications. Nat Biotechnol 2002;20:87–90.

15 Kaminuma O, Kitamura F, Miyatake S, Yamaoka K, Miyoshi H, Inokuma S, Tatsumi H, Nemoto S, Kitamura N, Mori A, Hiroi T: T-box 21 transcription factor is responsible for distorted T(H)2 differentiation in human peripheral CD4+ T cells. J Allergy Clin Immunol 2009;123:813 –823.e3.

16 Zhang DH, Yang L, Ray A: Differential responsiveness of the IL-5 and IL-4 genes to transcription factor GATA-3. J Immunol 1998;161:3817–3821.

17 Su RC, Becker AB, Kozyrskyj AL, Hayglass KT: Epigenetic regulation of established human type 1 versus type 2 cytokine responses. J Allergy Clin Immunol 2008;121:57–63.

18 Messi M, Giacchetto I, Nagata K, Lanzavecchia A, Natoli G, Sallusto F: Memory and flexibility of cytokine gene expression as separable properties of human T(H)1 and T(H)2 lymphocytes. Nat Immunol 2003;4:78–86.

19 Sundrud MS, Grill SM, Ni D, Nagata K, Alkan SS, Subramaniam A, Unutmaz D: Genetic reprogramming of primary human T cells reveals functional plasticity in Th cell differentiation. J Immunol 2003;171:3542–3549.

Original Paper

International Archives of Allergy and Immunology

Int Arch Allergy Immunol 2010;152(suppl 1):22–31
DOI: 10.1159/000312122

Published online: June 4, 2010

Prolonged Culture of Mast Cells with High-Glucose Medium Enhances the FcεRI-Mediated Degranulation Response and Leukotriene C_4 Production

Yuko Kitahata[a, b] Satoshi Nunomura[a] Tadashi Terui[b] Chisei Ra[a]

[a]Division of Molecular Cell Immunology and Allergology, Advanced Medical Research Center, and
[b]Department of Dermatology, Nihon University Graduate School of Medicine, Tokyo, Japan

Key Words
Degranulation · Eicosanoids · Glucose · Leukotrienes · Mast cells

Abstract
Background: Mast cell-released chemical mediators such as histamine, leukotriene (LT) C_4 and prostaglandin (PG) D_2 lead to the onset of allergic disorders. ATP provided from glycolysis is essential for histamine release and LTC_4 secretion from mast cells upon FcεRI cross-linking, indicating that glucose is a primary environmental factor for mast cell activation. In this study, we investigated whether increases in concentrations of glucose in culture media affect the activation of bone marrow-derived mouse mast cells (BMMCs) upon FcεRI cross-linking. ***Methods:*** BMMCs were cultured in RPMI-1640 supplemented with varying concentrations (5.5, 11, 16.5, 22, 27.5 and 33 mM) of D-glucose for 3 h, or 1, 3 or 7 days. D-Mannitol was added to the medium containing 5.5 mM D-glucose for osmotic control. After culturing, these cells were sensitized with anti-TNP IgE and then stimulated with TNP-BSA. ***Results:*** We found that long-term culture (7 days) of BMMCs with 33 mM D-glucose increases the FcεRI-dependent release of β-hexosaminidase and LTC_4 without affecting surface expression levels of FcεRI, intracellular ATP levels or calcium signaling. Biochemical analyses demonstrated that FcεRI-dependent phosphorylation of cytosolic phospholipase A_2 ($cPLA_2$) at the Ser505 residue was significantly increased by culturing with 33 mM glucose. ***Conclusions:*** Taken together, our data suggest that glucose can augment FcεRI-mediated mast cell activation, particularly the degranulation response and LTC_4 secretion after prolonged culture of mast cells with high-glucose medium. Moreover, it is suggested that increased phosphorylation of $cPLA_2$ at the Ser505 residue contributes to the enhancement of LTC_4 secretion.

Introduction

Mast cells express the high-affinity receptors for IgE (FcεRI), which are comprised of an IgE-binding α-chain and two types of signaling subunits, a β-chain and a disulfide-linked homodimer of γ-chains [1]. Upon FcεRI engagement, mast cells immediately release inflammatory mediators such as histamine, leukotriene (LT) C_4 and prostaglandin (PG) D_2, which in turn lead to the development of allergic disorders [2].

KARGER

Fax +41 61 306 12 34
E-Mail karger@karger.ch
www.karger.com

1018–2438/10/1525–0022$26.00/0

Accessible online at:
www.karger.com/iaa

Correspondence to: Dr. Chisei Ra, Division of Molecular
Cell Immunology and Allergology, Advanced Medical Research Center
Nihon University Graduate School of Medical Science
30-1 Oyaguchikami-cho, Itabashi-ku, Tokyo 173-8610 (Japan)
Tel. +81 3 3972 8111, Fax +81 3 3972 8227, E-Mail fcericra@med.nihon-u.ac.jp

Previous studies suggested that glucose deficiency results in a rapid reduction in intracellular ATP production and causes the inhibition of histamine release and LTC_4 secretion by mast cells upon FcεRI cross-linking [3, 4]. These findings suggest that glucose metabolism plays an important biological role in FcεRI-mediated mast cell activation. In addition, it was reported that increased glucose levels up-regulate the catalytic activity of cytosolic phospholipase A_2 ($cPLA_2$) [5–8], the expression of cyclooxygenases (COXs) and lipoxygenases (LOXs) [9–12], and the concentration of intracellular calcium $[Ca^{2+}]_i$ [13–15] in various types of mammalian cells. In general, $cPLA_2$ generates arachidonic acid from membrane lipids, and LOXs and COXs further convert the arachidonic acid into LTs and PGs, respectively [16]. Other previous studies indicated that intracellular calcium signaling is indispensable for both histamine release and eicosanoid secretion in mast cells [2]. Collectively, these findings suggest that increases in glucose levels may augment mast cell activation following FcεRI engagement.

In the present study, we investigated the effects of increased glucose concentrations on FcεRI-mediated mast cell activation by monitoring the degranulation response and eicosanoid production in bone marrow-derived mouse mast cells (BMMCs).

Materials and Methods

Reagents

Anti-TNP IgE mAb (clone IgE3) was purchased from BD PharMingen (San Diego, Calif., USA) and labeled with Alexa488 (Molecular Probe/Invitrogen, Tokyo, Japan). Glucose-free RPMI-1640 medium (11879020) was purchased from Invitrogen. TNP-BSA (25 mol of TNP/mol of BSA) was purchased from LSL (Tokyo, Japan). Recombinant murine IL-3 was purchased from PeproTech (Rocky Hill, NJ, USA). D-Mannitol and a PKH67 Green Fluorescent Cell Linker Kit were purchased from Sigma (St. Louis, Mo., USA). Intracellular ATP determination kit and D-glucose were purchased from Wako Chemical (Tokyo, Japan). Polyclonal antibodies against $cPLA_2$ and phosphorylated $cPLA_2$ were purchased from Cell Signaling Technology (Beverly, Mass., USA).

Preparation of BMMCs

Following approval by the Committee of Animal Care and Use of the Nihon University, BMMCs were prepared from the femurs of 4- to 8-week-old C57BL/6J mice as described previously [17] and used for experiments after 4–5 weeks of culture.

Treatment of BMMCs with Glucose

D-Glucose (5.5, 11, 16.5, 22, 27.5 and 33 mM) was added to glucose-free RPMI-1640 medium (11879020, Invitrogen) containing IL-3 (4 ng/ml). BMMCs (2×10^6) were cultured in 10 ml of RPMI-1640 medium for 3 h, or 1, 3 or 7 days. In the 7-day culture, the medium was exchanged every other day. A sample with 5.5 mM D-glucose was used as the normal control. D-Mannitol was added to the culture medium containing 5.5 mM D-glucose as the osmotic control.

Degranulation Assay

The degranulation response was evaluated by β-hexosaminidase release. IgE-sensitized BMMCs (2×10^5/ml) were stimulated with or without 0.3, 1 or 10 ng/ml TNP-BSA at 37°C for 30 min in 0.2 ml of 1× Tyrode's buffer. The supernatants were collected, and the β-hexosaminidase activity in the supernatant was determined as previously described [17]. Cell extracts lysed with 0.1% Triton X-100 were used to quantify the total β-hexosaminidase activity. The percentage of net β-hexosaminidase release was calculated as follows: (supernatant optical density of the stimulated cells – supernatant optical density of the unstimulated cells) × 100/(the total cell lysate optical density of unstimulated cells – supernatant optical density value of unstimulated cells).

Measurement of LTC_4 and PGD_2

IgE-sensitized BMMCs (2×10^5/ml) were stimulated with or without TNP-BSA at the indicated concentrations for 30 min in 0.2 ml of 1× Tyrode's buffer. The supernatants after FcεRI stimulation were analyzed with specific EIA kits (Cayman Chemical, Ann Arbor, Mich., USA).

Measurement of IL-6

IgE-sensitized BMMCs (2×10^5/ml) were stimulated with or without 1 ng/ml TNP-BSA for 6 h in 0.2 ml of RPMI-1640 supplemented with 2% (v/v) FBS. The production of IL-6 was analyzed with a specific ELISA kit (BioSource International, Camarillo, Calif., USA)

Flow Cytometry

To evaluate FcεRI expression at the cell surface, BMMCs (2×10^5) were labeled with 1 μg/ml of Alexa488-conjugated anti-TNP IgE at 4°C for 30 min in 0.1 ml of PBS containing 0.1% sodium azide and then washed twice with the same buffer. The cells were analyzed with FACSCalibur (Becton-Dickinson Biosciences, San Jose, Calif., USA). For detecting apoptotic cells, the cells (1×10^5) were double stained with annexin V-fluorescein isothiocyanate (FITC) and propidium iodide (PI) for 15 min at room temperature and then analyzed employing the FACSCalibur. Double-negative cells (annexin V-FITC–/PI–) were considered to be viable cells. In some experiments, BMMCs (2×10^5) were labeled with a PKH67 green fluorescent cell linker kit (Sigma) to analyze cell division.

Measurement of $[Ca^{2+}]_i$ Mobilization

The IgE-sensitized cells (1×10^6) were loaded with 4 μM Fluo3-AM (Dojindo, Kumamoto, Japan) for 30 min at 37°C. The cells were resuspended in 1× Tyrode's buffer, and then changes in dye fluorescence upon the addition of TNP-BSA were monitored employing flow cytometry. $[Ca^{2+}]_i$ mobilization was expressed as the relative fluorescence intensity.

Immunoblotting

The stimulated cells (5×10^6) were washed twice with ice-cold PBS and lysed in Tris-buffered saline containing 1% Nonidet P-40, 2 mM phenylmethylsulfonylfluoride, 10 μg/ml aprotinin, 2 μg/ml leupeptin and pepstatin A, 50 mM NaF and 1 mM sodium orthovanadate for 30 min on ice. The lysates were centrifuged for 20 min at 14,000 *g*. The samples were then boiled, separated by 10% SDS-PAGE and transferred to an Immobilon-P membrane (Millipore, Bedford, Mass., USA). The membrane was incubated with primary antibody and an appropriate secondary horseradish peroxidase-conjugated antibody. Signals were detected by enhanced chemiluminescence (GE Healthcare Bio-sciences, Little Chalfont, UK). The immunoreactive bands were scanned to produce digital images that were quantified employing Scion Image software, and then x-fold phosphorylation was calculated from the amount of phosphoprotein relative to the corresponding non-phospho-loading control.

RT-PCR

Total RNA was isolated from BMMCs using ISOGEN (Nippon Gene, Tokyo, Japan). cDNA was reverse transcribed from 2 μg of total RNA with 200 U of SuperScriptII, 2.5 mM dNTP and 1.0 mM oligo(dT) primer. The resultant cDNA was then employed as templates for PCR. The open reading frames of β-actin, 5-LOX, COX-1 and COX-2 were amplified using appropriate primers as follows: 5′-ATGGATGACGATACGCTGC-3′ and 5′-CCATCACAATG-CCTGTGGTA-3′ (β-actin); 5′-TGGCTCCATGATGACTGGTA-3′ and 5′-ACTCTCTCCAGGGGTTTGGT-3′ (5-LOX); 5′-GA-AGGAGTCTCTCGCTCTGG-3′ and 5′-CTGGTGGGTGAAG-TGTTGTG-3′ (COX-1); 5′-AAACCGTGGGGAATGTATGA-3′ and 5′-AGTGTCTTTGACTGTGGGGG-3′ (COX-2). PCR was performed as follows: denaturation at 94°C for 30 s, annealing at 60°C for 30 s and extension at 72°C for 1 min. The PCR products were resolved on a 1% agarose gel and visualized by ethidium bromide staining. The visualized bands were scanned to produce digital images that were quantified employing Scion Image software, and then x-fold increase was calculated from the intensity of bands in cells cultured in high-glucose medium or in osmotic control medium relative to the intensity of bands in cells cultured with 5.5 mM D-glucose.

Statistical Analysis

The data shown are means ± SD. One-way ANOVA was used to test for differences among multiple groups. Statistical significances between two groups were analyzed using Student's t test; $p < 0.05$ was considered significant.

Results

Prolonged Culture in High-Glucose Medium Amplifies the FcεRI-Dependent Degranulation Response of Mast Cells

First, we examined whether increases in D-glucose concentrations (5.5, 11, 22 or 33 mM) of culture medium affect the mast cell degranulation response induced by IgE and antigen (1 ng/ml). As shown in figure 1a, enhancement of the FcεRI-mediated release of β-hexosaminidase was observed 3 h, and 1 and 7 days after culture. However, the culture of BMMCs in the osmotic control medium (5.5 mM D-glucose + D-mannitol) for 3 h or 1 day also increased the FcεRI-dependent degranulation response. The culture of cells in the medium supplemented with 33 mM D-glucose for 7 days induced osmolarity-independent augmentation of β-hexosaminidase release. Figure 1b shows that culturing with 27.5 mM D-glucose for 7 days failed to increase the release of β-hexosaminidase. Slight augmentation of the FcεRI-mediated degranulation response was seen when BMMCs were cultured with 30 mM D-glucose (data not shown).

Prolonged Culture in High-Glucose Medium Amplifies FcεRI-Dependent LTC_4 Secretion of Mast Cells

Next, we examined whether prolonged culture of BMMCs in high-glucose medium (33 mM) enhances FcεRI-mediated secretion of LTC_4. BMMCs were cultured in medium containing D-glucose (5.5, 11, 22, 27.5 or 33 mM) or with the osmotic control medium (5.5 mM D-glucose + D-mannitol) for 7 days. As with the degranulation response, the secretion of LTC_4 was increased by prolonged culture in 33 mM D-glucose (fig. 2a). Furthermore, we examined the effects of prolonged culture in 33 mM D-glucose on the production of PGD_2 and IL-6 induced by FcεRI stimulation. Figure 2b shows that increased concentrations of D-glucose and D-mannitol amplified the secretion of PGD_2, suggesting that PGD_2 secretion was enhanced in an osmolarity-dependent fashion. On the other hand, the production of IL-6 following FcεRI stimulation was unaltered even when BMMCs were cultured in 33 mM D-glucose or in the osmotic control medium (fig. 2c).

Mast Cells Cultured in High-Glucose Medium Show an Increased Degranulation Response and LTC_4 Release in Response to Different Antigen Concentrations

As demonstrated in figures 1 and 2, prolonged culture of mast cells in high-glucose medium (33 mM) increases β-hexosaminidase release and LTC_4 secretion induced by IgE and 1 ng/ml antigen. We further examined whether the augmentation of β-hexosaminidase release and LTC_4 secretion of mast cells differed in response to antigen concentrations. To address this issue, FcεRI was engaged with IgE and 0.3 or 10 ng/ml antigen. Under the above experimental conditions, the degranulation response was reduced compared to BMMCs stimulated with IgE and 1 ng/ml of antigen (fig. 3a). On the other hand, comparable levels of LTC_4 were released from BMMCs stimulated with 0.3, 1 or 10 ng/ml antigen (fig. 3b). Figure 3 shows that prolonged culture of BMMCs in high-glucose medium enhanced the degranulation response and LTC_4 secretion induced by 0.3, 1 or 10 ng/ml antigen.

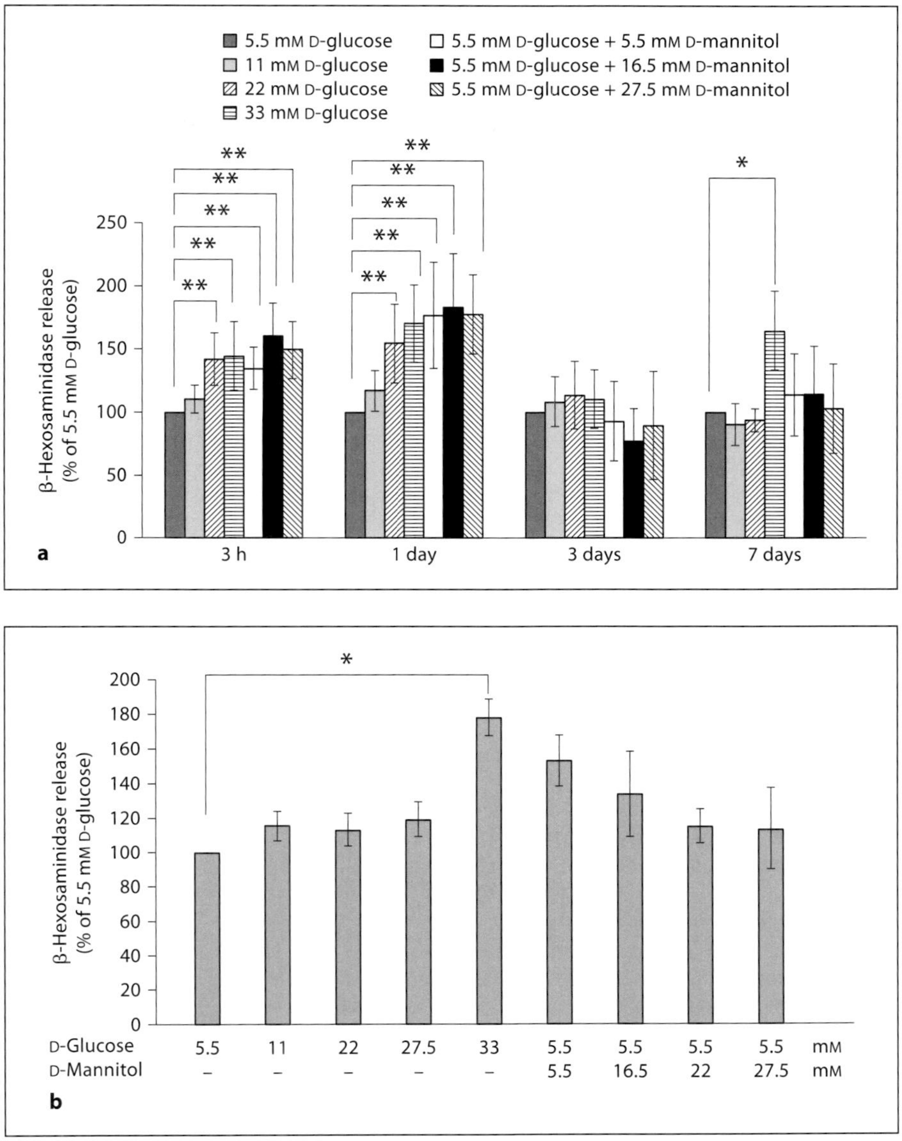

Fig. 1. Amplifying effects of long-term culture of BMMCs in high-glucose medium on FcεRI-dependent release of β-hexosaminidase. **a** BMMCs (2×10^5/ml) were cultured in medium containing D-glucose (5.5, 11, 16.5, 22 or 33 mM) or in the osmotic control medium (5.5 mM D-glucose + D-mannitol) for 3 h, or 1, 3 or 7 days. **b** BMMCs (2×10^5/ml) were cultured in medium containing D-glucose (5.5, 11, 16.5, 22, 27.5 or 33 mM) or in the osmotic control medium (5.5 mM D-glucose + D-mannitol) for 7 days. After culture, these cells were sensitized with anti-TNP IgE and then stimulated with 1 ng/ml TNP-BSA for 30 min. The degranulation assay was performed as described in Materials and Methods. The FcεRI-triggered net release of β-hexosaminidase from BMMCs cultured in 5.5 mM D-glucose was expressed as 100%. **a** The net release of β-hexosaminidase from BMMCs cultured in 5.5 mM D-glucose was 32.0 ± 1.9 (3 h), 26.3 ± 1.3 (1 day), 23.1 ± 1.6 (3 days) and 30.0 ± 0.5% (7 days). **b** The net release of β-hexosaminidase by BMMCs cultured in 5.5 mM D-glucose was 32.9 ± 2.9%. Means ± SD of triplicate samples. Similar results were obtained from three independent experiments. Student's t test: * $p < 0.05$, ** $p < 0.01$.

Cell Surface FcεRI Expression, Intracellular ATP Levels and Cell Viability of Mast Cells Are Not Altered by Long-Term Culture in High-Glucose Medium

To clarify the molecular mechanisms involved in the amplification of the degranulation response and LTC_4 secretion, we examined the surface expression of FcεRI. BMMCs were cultured in medium containing D-glucose (5.5 or 33 mM) or in the osmotic control medium (5.5 mM D-glucose + 27.5 mM D-mannitol) for 7 days. As shown in figure 4a, prolonged culture of BMMCs with 33 mM D-glucose failed to increase the levels of cell surface FcεRI expression. Since preformed-chemical mediators and LTC_4 are released from mast cells in an energy-dependent manner [3, 4], we next examined the levels of intracellular ATP. Figure 4b shows that levels of intracellular ATP were not altered by prolonged culture in 33 mM D-glucose. In relation to these observations, long-term culture of BMMCs with 33 mM D-glucose had no effect on cell division, growth or viability (fig. 5).

Prolonged Culture of BMMCs in High-Glucose Medium Fails to Increase FcεRI-Dependent Calcium Mobilization

Previous studies reported that D-glucose affects $[Ca^{2+}]_i$ levels [13–15]. In addition, $[Ca^{2+}]_i$ is an essential second messenger for chemical mediator release [18, 19]. Thus,

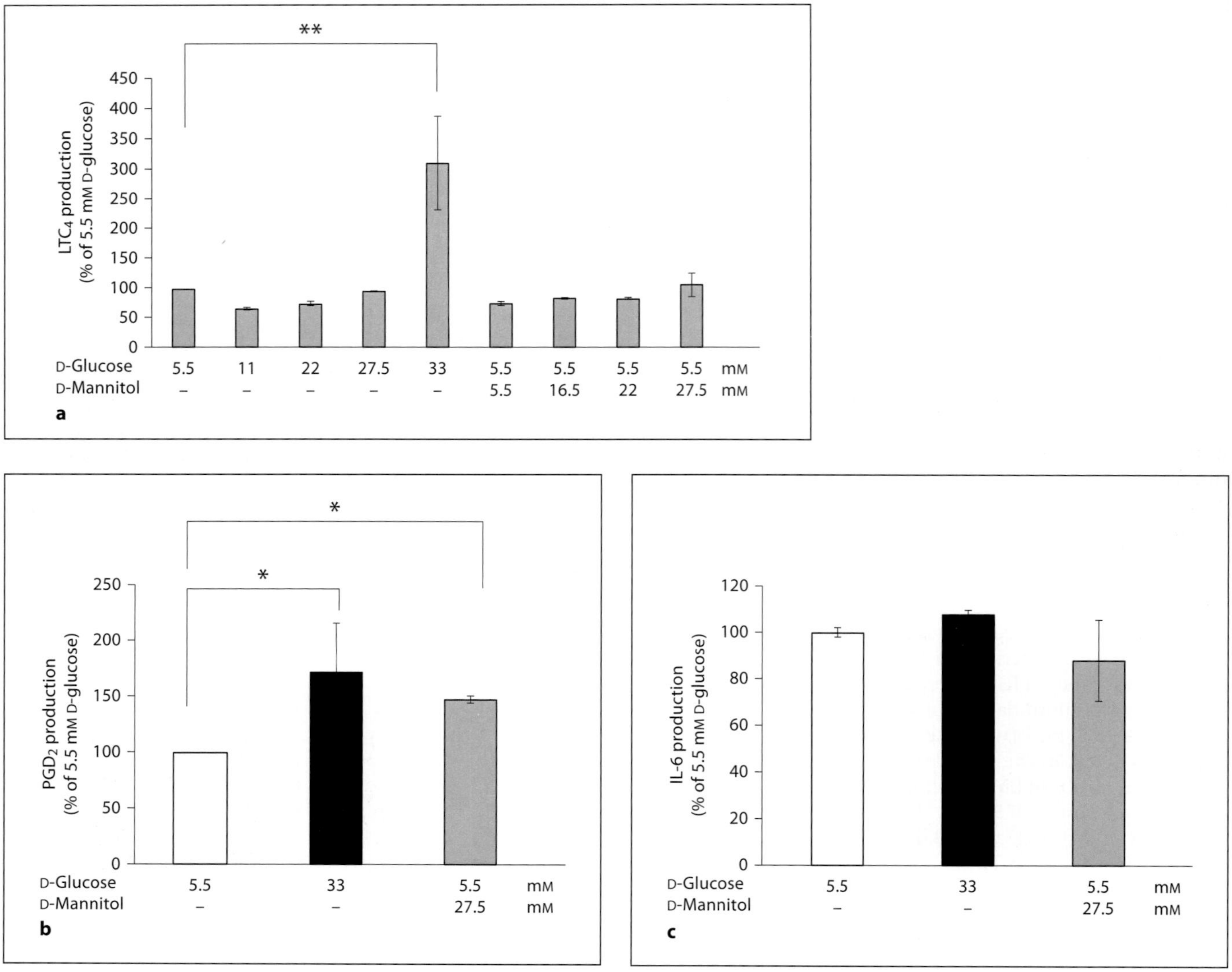

Fig. 2. Amplifying effects of long-term culture of BMMCs in high-glucose medium on FcεRI-dependent LTC_4 secretion. **a** BMMCs (2×10^5/ml) were cultured in medium containing D-glucose (5.5, 11, 22, 27.5 or 33 mM) or in the osmotic control medium (5.5 mM D-glucose + D-mannitol) for 7 days. After culture, these cells were sensitized with anti-TNP IgE and then stimulated with 1 ng/ml TNP-BSA for 30 min. LTC_4 secretion was measured by a specific EIA kit. **b** BMMCs (2×10^5/ml) were cultured in medium containing D-glucose (5.5 or 33 mM) or in the osmotic control medium (5.5 mM D-glucose + 27.5 mM D-mannitol) for 7 days. IgE-sensitized cells were stimulated with 1 ng/ml of TNP-BSA as in **a**. PGD_2 secretion was measured using a specific EIA kit. **c** BMMCs (2×10^6) were cultured with D-glucose as in **b**. IgE-sensitized cells were stimulated with 1 ng/ml TNP-BSA for 6 h. IL-6 production was measured by a specific ELISA kit. **a–c** The FcεRI-triggered net release of eicosanoids and IL-6 from BMMCs cultured in 5.5 mM D-glucose was expressed as 100%. The net release of LTC_4, PGD_2 and IL-6 was 304.5 ± 46.3, 11.7 ± 6.1 and 176.2 ± 16.3 ng/ml, respectively. Means ± SD of triplicate samples. Similar results were obtained from three independent experiments. Student's t test: * $p < 0.05$, ** $p < 0.01$.

we examined the effects of prolonged culture in high-glucose medium (33 mM) on $[Ca^{2+}]_i$ mobilization triggered by FcεRI stimulation. BMMCs were cultured in medium containing D-glucose (5.5 or 33 mM) or in the osmotic control medium (5.5 mM D-glucose + 27.5 mM D-mannitol) for 7 days. As shown in figure 6, engagement of FcεRI with IgE and 1 ng/ml antigen, or stimulation with calcium ionophore induced apparent mobilization of $[Ca^{2+}]_i$ in all three groups. However, no significant difference in the levels of $[Ca^{2+}]_i$ mobilization was observed among the three groups.

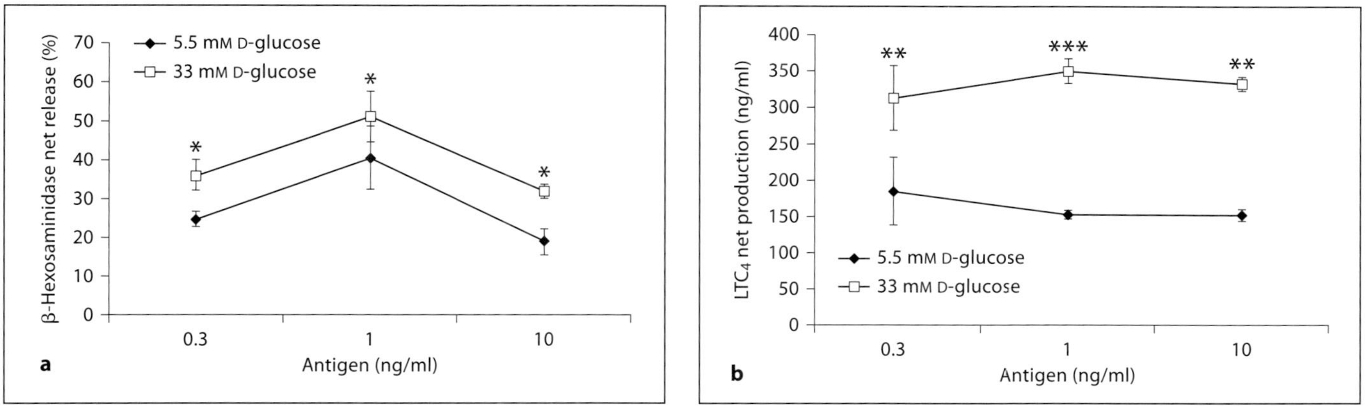

Fig. 3. BMMCs cultured in high-glucose medium show an increased degranulation response and LTC_4 release in response to different antigen concentrations. BMMCs (2 × 10^5/ml) were cultured in medium containing D-glucose (5.5 or 33 mM) or in the osmotic control medium (5.5 mM D-glucose + 27.5 mM D-mannitol) for 7 days. After culture, these cells were sensitized with anti-TNP IgE and then stimulated with 0.3, 1 or 10 ng/ml TNP-BSA for 30 min. **a** FcεRI-triggered net release of β-hexosaminidase. **b** FcεRI-triggered net production of LTC_4. Means ± SD of triplicate samples. Similar results were obtained from three independent experiments. Student's t test: * $p < 0.05$, ** $p < 0.01$, *** $p < 0.001$, vs. cells treated with 33 mM D-glucose.

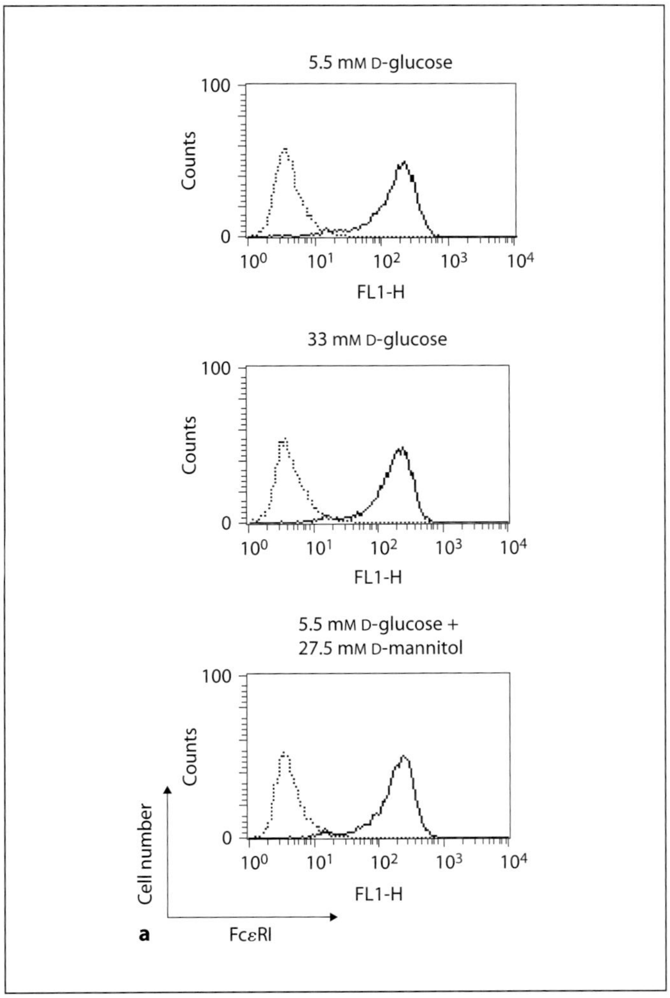

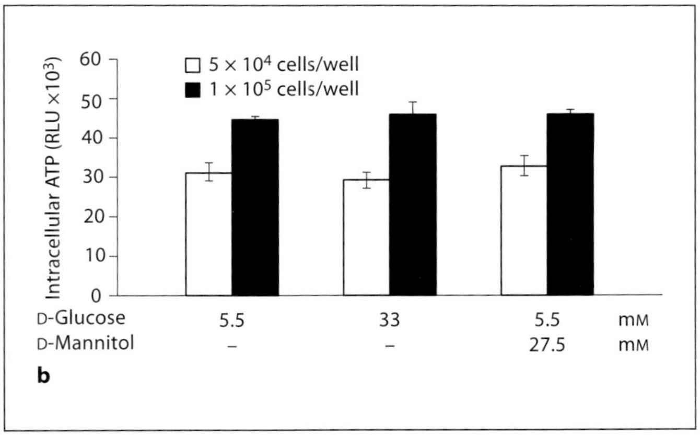

Fig. 4. Prolonged exposure of BMMCs to high-glucose medium has no effects on cell surface FcεRI expression or intracellular ATP levels. BMMCs (2 × 10^5/ml) were cultured in medium containing D-glucose (5.5 or 33 mM) or in the osmotic control medium (5.5 mM D-glucose + 27.5 mM D-mannitol) for 7 days. **a** FcεRI expression on the cell surface was analyzed using a flow cytometer. The results shown are representative of three independent experiments with similar results. **b** Intracellular ATP levels were measured employing a luciferase-based intracellular ATP measurement kit. Means ± SD of samples obtained from three independent experiments. No significant difference was observed (Student's t test).

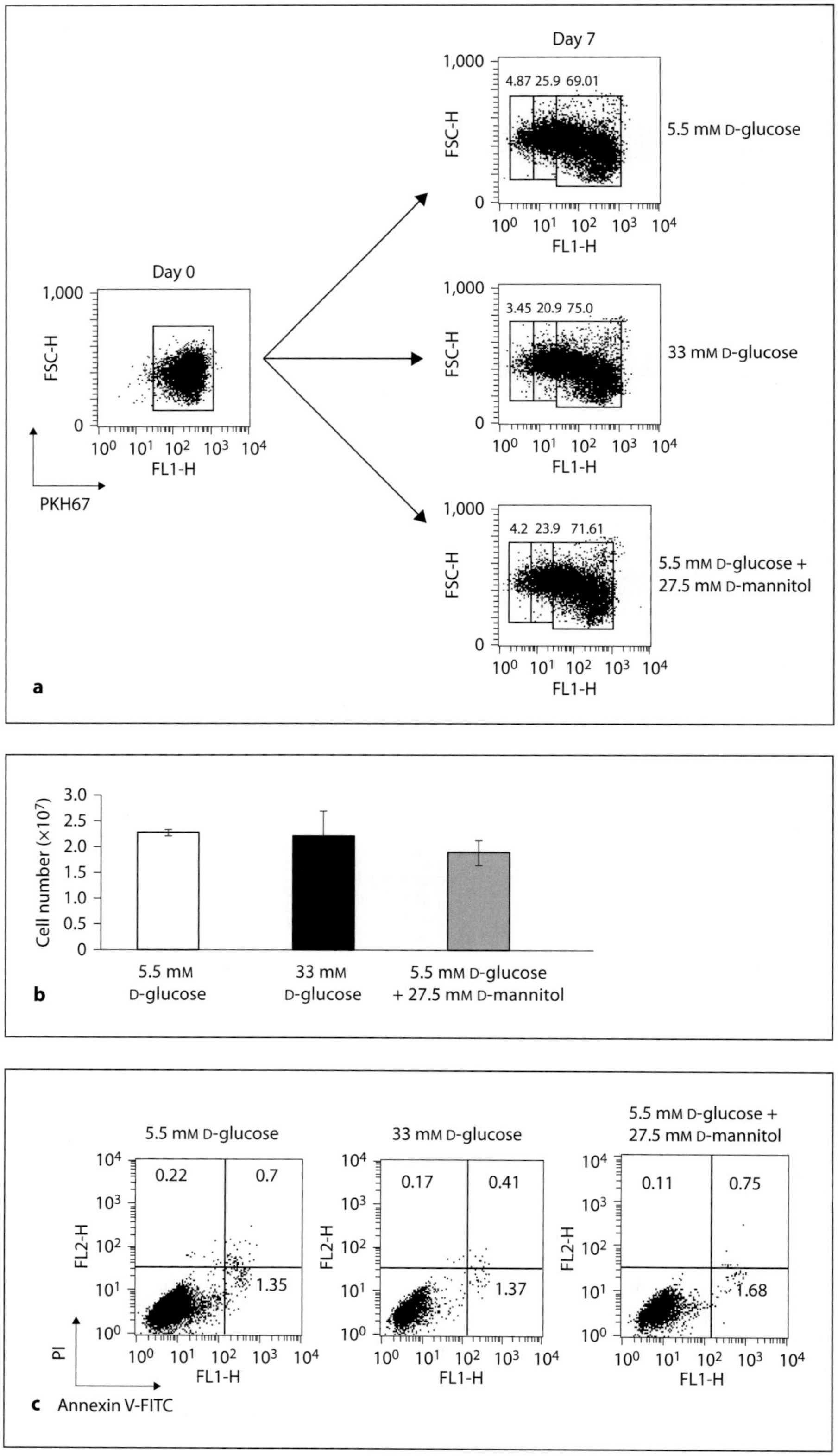

Fig. 5. Prolonged exposure of BMMCs to high-glucose medium has no effects on cell growth or cell viability. BMMCs (2×10^5/ml) were cultured in medium containing D-glucose (5.5 or 33 mM) or in the osmotic control medium (5.5 mM D-glucose + 27.5 mM D-mannitol) for 7 days. **a** Cell division was evaluated by decreases in intensities of PKH67 fluorescence dye. **b** The total cell number was evaluated. Means ± SD of samples obtained from three independent experiments. Student's t test was performed between the cells treated with 5.5 mM D-glucose and the other cells. **c** The cells (1×10^5) were double stained with annexin V-FITC and PI. Double-negative cells (annexin V-FITC–/PI–) were considered to be viable cells. **a**, **c** The results shown are representative of three independent experiments with similar results.

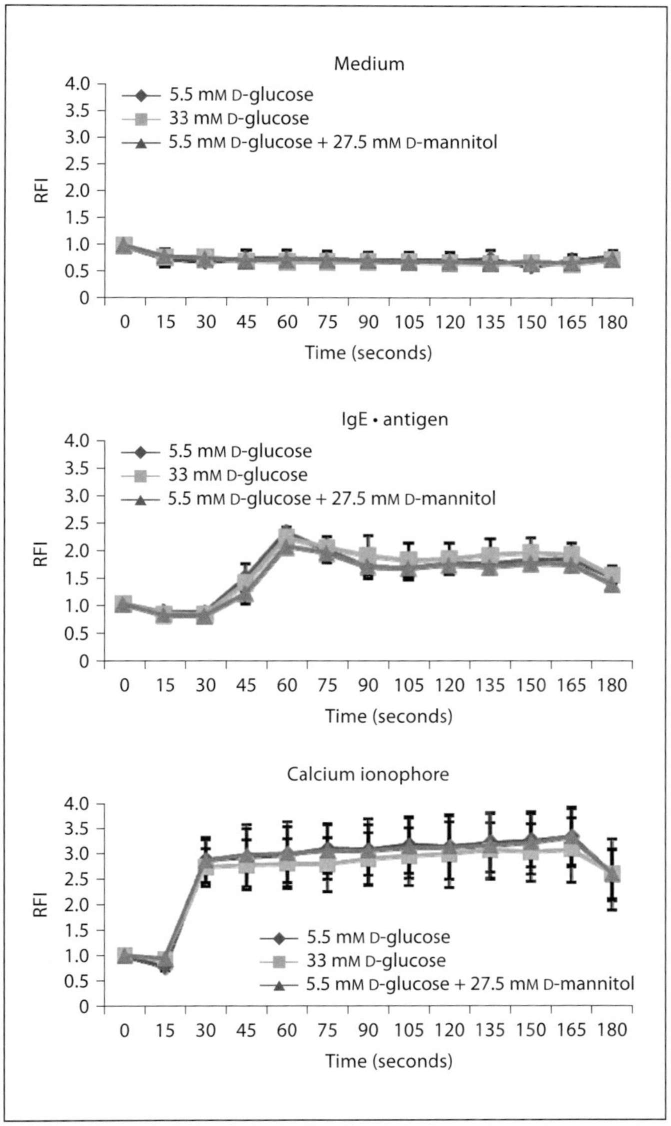

Fig. 6. Prolonged culture of BMMCs in high-glucose medium fails to increase FcεRI-dependent calcium mobilization. BMMCs (2×10^5/ml) were cultured in medium containing D-glucose (5.5 or 33 mM) or in the osmotic control medium (5.5 mM D-glucose + 27.5 mM D-mannitol) for 7 days. These cells were sensitized with anti-TNP IgE, and then the cells were incubated with 4 μM Fluo-3-AM for 20 min at 37°C. Changes in dye fluorescence were determined employing flow cytometry after stimulation with TNP-BSA at the indicated concentrations. $[Ca^{2+}]_i$ mobilization was expressed as the relative fluorescence intensity (RFI). A23187 was used as the positive control. Means ± SD of samples obtained from three independent experiments. Student's t test was performed between the cells treated with 5.5 mM D-glucose and the other cells.

FcεRI-Dependent Ser505 Phosphorylation of $cPLA_2$ Is Enhanced in BMMCs Cultured with High-Glucose Medium

To clarify the amplifying effects of prolonged culture with high glucose (33 mM) on LTC_4 release, we examined the metabolic cascade involving arachidonic acid. Phosphorylation of $cPLA_2$ at Ser505 is necessary for the release of arachidonic acid from the cell membrane in various types of cells [20–23]. BMMCs were cultured in medium containing D-glucose (5.5 or 33 mM) or in the osmotic control medium (5.5 mM D-glucose + 27.5 mM D-mannitol) for 7 days. Figure 7a shows that Ser505 of $cPLA_2$ was spontaneously phosphorylated and that the level of phosphorylation was increased upon cross-linking of FcεRI with IgE and antigen (1 ng/ml). FcεRI-mediated Ser505 phosphorylation of $cPLA_2$ in BMMCs was enhanced by the culture with 33 mM D-glucose (1.6 times). Moreover, we investigated whether expression levels of 5-LOX, COX-1 and COX-2 mRNA changed among the three groups (5.5 mM D-glucose, 33 mM D-glucose, 5.5 mM D-glucose + 27.5 mM D-mannitol). As shown in figure 7b, neither high glucose nor mannitol affected 5-LOX mRNA expression. COX-2 expression was undetectable in all groups. On the other hand, COX-1 mRNA expression was strongly or slightly increased in BMMCs cultured in medium containing 33 mM D-glucose or in the osmotic control medium, respectively.

Discussion

In this study, we found that culture of mast cells in high-glucose medium for 7 days augments FcεRI-mediated β-hexosaminidase release and LTC_4 secretion in an osmolarity-independent manner (fig. 1, 2). In contrast, no significant effects of high-glucose medium on the above responses were observed in mast cells cultured for 3 days. This is the first report demonstrating novel roles of glucose in FcεRI-dependent mast cell activation. It is worth noting that mast cells cultured under high-glucose conditions show an increased degranulation response to suboptimal antigen concentration (0.3 ng/ml) as well as optimal antigen concentration (1 ng/ml; fig. 3). This finding suggests that prolonged culture of mast cells in high-glucose conditions may increase the sensitivity of mast cells to low-dose antigen.

Although the prolonged culture effectively increased both the secretion of LTC_4 and the release of β-hexosaminidase, the same treatment did not enhance cell surface FcεRI expression, levels of intracellular ATP or

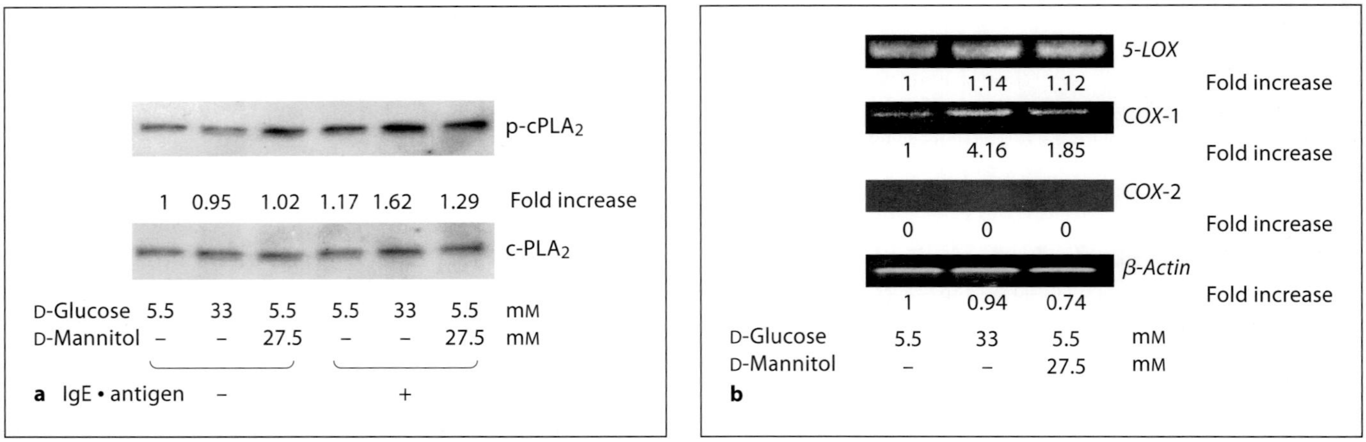

Fig. 7. BMMCs cultured in high-glucose medium show increased phosphorylation on Ser505 of $cPLA_2$ upon FcεRI stimulation. BMMCs (2×10^5/ml) were cultured in medium containing D-glucose (5.5 or 33 mM) or in the osmotic control medium (5.5 mM D-glucose + 27.5 mM D-mannitol) for 7 days. **a** These cells were sensitized with anti-TNP IgE and then stimulated with or without 1 ng/ml TNP-BSA for 1 min. Total cell lysates were analyzed by immunoblotting with anti-phospho $cPLA_2$ (Ser505) antibody, and the blot was reprobed with anti-$cPLA_2$ antibody. **b** After culture, total RNA was prepared and analyzed for transcription levels of *COX-1, COX-2,* and *5-LOX* genes by RT-PCR. The housekeeping gene encoding *β-actin* was employed as internal control. The results shown are representative of three independent experiments with similar results. **a, b** The intensities of the bands were expressed as fold increases relative to the intensity of bands observed in cells cultured with 5.5 mM D-glucose.

$[Ca^{2+}]_i$ mobilization (fig. 4–6). Thus, we could not elucidate the mechanisms responsible for the augmentation of the degranulation response in the present study. We speculate that S-D-lactoylglutathione, an intermediate product of the glycolysis side pathway, participates in the amplification. This is suggested because (i) mast cells abundantly express an enzyme to generate S-D-lactoylglutathione from D-glucose [24], (ii) S-D-lactoylglutathione induces microtubule formation [25], which is an indispensable process for the degranulation response [26, 27], and (iii) IgE-dependent histamine release from human peripheral leukocytes is augmented upon loading of S-D-lactoylglutathione [25].

In regard to enhanced LTC_4 secretion, we demonstrated that Ser505 phosphorylation of $cPLA_2$ in mast cells cultured with high-glucose medium was maximally increased upon FcεRI stimulation (fig. 7a). Since the degree of $cPLA_2$ Ser505 phosphorylation shows a good correlation with its enzymatic activity [23], we concluded that the modification in levels of $cPLA_2$ phosphorylation, at least in part, is responsible for the glucose-mediated enhancement of LTC_4 secretion.

In addition to Ser505 phosphorylation of $cPLA_2$, the expression of COX-1 mRNA was significantly up-regulated in mast cells after long-term culture with high-glucose (fig. 7b). These up-regulations might have amplifying effects on FcεRI-dependent PGD_2 secretion (fig. 2b). However, we observed comparable enhancement of PGD_2 secretion from mast cells cultured with the osmotic control medium (fig. 2b). In mast cells cultured in the osmotic control medium, expression levels of COX-1 mRNA were slightly increased compared to the control cells, but the level was much less than that of the cells cultured in high-glucose medium. Thus, we believe that other unknown mechanisms contribute to increased PGD_2 production by mast cells cultured with the osmotic control medium, although we cannot exclude the involvement of up-regulated COX-1 expression.

Augmentation of FcεRI-dependent mast cell activation by glucose was observed at 33 mM. However, it seems that this concentration is much higher than that of the physiological glucose concentration in blood. In case glucose alters mast cell activation in response to FcεRI-independent stimulants such as neuropeptides at concentrations <33 mM, comparison between the present and such studies would be useful for elucidation of glucose-mediated effects on mast cell activation.

In conclusion, the findings of the present study suggest that glucose acts as a regulating factor for the FcεRI-mediated degranulation response and LTC_4 secretion. However, the mechanisms underlying the enhancing effects of glucose on the degranulation response remain unclear. We are currently investigating the roles of S-D-lactoylglutathione in this process.

Acknowledgment

This work was supported by the grants-in-aid for private universities from the Ministry of Education, Culture, Sports, Science and Technology of Japan.

Disclosure Statement

The authors declare that no financial or other conflict of interest exists in relation to the content of this article.

References

1 Ra C, Jouvin MH, Kinet JP: Complete structure of the mouse mast cell receptor for IgE (Fc epsilon RI) and surface expression of chimeric receptors (rat-mouse-human) on transfected cells. J Biol Chem 1989;264:15323–15327.
2 Gilfillan AM, Rivera J: The tyrosine kinase network regulating mast cell activation. Immunol Rev 2009;228:149–169.
3 Takei M, Endo K: Histamine release and calcium concentrations in rat mast cells are dependent on intracellular ATP: effects of prostaglandin D_2. Prostaglandins Leukot Essential Fatty Acids 1994;50:357–362.
4 Nguyen T, Gupta S: Leukotriene C_4 secretion from normal murine mast cells by a probenecid-sensitive and multidrug resistance-associated protein-independent mechanism. J Immunol 1997;158:4916 -4920.
5 Haneda M, Araki S, Togawa M, Sugimoto T, Isono M, Kikkawa R: Mitogen-activated protein kinase cascade is activated in glomeruli of diabetic rats and glomerular mesangial cells cultured under high glucose conditions. Diabetes 1997;46:847–853.
6 Hayama M, Akiba S, Fukuzumi M, Sato T: High glucose-induced cytosolic phospholipase A2 activation responsible for eicosanoid production in rat mesangial cells. J Biochem 1997;122:1196–1201.
7 Kim YH, Han HJ: High-glucose-induced prostaglandin E(2) and peroxisome proliferator-activated receptor delta promote mouse embryonic stem cell proliferation. Stem Cells 2008;26:745–755.
8 Dunlop M, Clark S: Glucose-induced phosphorylation and activation of high molecular weight cytosolic phospholipase A2 in neonatal rat pancreatic islets. J Biochem Cell Biol 1995;27:1191–1199.
9 Shanmugum N, Gaw Gonzolo IT, Natarajan R: Molecular mechanism of high glucose-induced cyclooxygenase-2 expression in monocytes. Diabetes 2004;53:795–802.
10 Sheu ML, Ho FM, Chao KF, Kuo ML, Liu SH: Activation of phosphoinositide 3-kinase in response to high glucose leads to regulation of reactive oxygen species-related nuclear factor-κB activation and cyclooxygenase-2 expression in mesangial cells. Mol Pharmacol 2004;66:187–196.
11 Kang SW, Adler SG, Nast CC, Lapage J, Gu JT, Nadler JL, Natarajan R: 12-Lipoxygenase is increased in glucose-stimulated mesangial cells and in experimental diabetic nephropathy. Kidney Int 2001;59:1354–1362.
12 Kim YS, Xu ZG, Reddy MA, Li SL, Lanting L, Sharma K, Adler SG , Natarajan R: Novel interactions between TGF-β1 actions and the 12/15-lipoxygenase pathway in mesangial cells. J Am Soc Nephrol 2005;16:352–362.
13 Liu D, Maier A, Scholze A, Rauch U, Boltzen U, Zhao Z, Zhu Z, Tepel M: High glucose enhances transient receptor potential channel canonical type 6-dependent calcium influx in human platelets via phosphatidylinositol 3-kinase-dependent pathway. Arterioscler Thromb Vasc Biol 2008;28:746–751.
14 Trus M, Corkey RF, Nesher R, Richard AM, Deeney JT, Corkey BE, Atlas D: The L-type voltage-gated Ca^{2+} channel is the Ca^{2+} sensor protein of stimulus-secretion coupling in pancreatic beta cells. Biochemistry 2007;46:14461–11467.
15 Song JH, Jung SY, Hong SB, Kim MJ, Suh CK: Effect of high glucose on basal intracellular calcium regulation in rat mesangial cell. Am J Nephrol 2003;23:343–352.
16 Boyce JA: Mast cells and eicosanoid mediators: a system of reciprocal paracrine and autocrine regulation. Immunol Rev 2007;217:168–185.
17 Nunomura S, Gon Y, Yoshimaru T, Suzuki Y, Nishimoto H, Kawakami T, Ra C: Role of the FcεRI beta-chain ITAM as a signal regulator for mast cell activation with monomeric IgE. Int Immunol 2005;17:685–694.
18 Gijón MA, Leslie CC: Regulation of arachidonic acid release and cytosolic phospholipase A2 activation. J Leukoc Biol 1999;65:330–336.
19 Di Capite J, Parekh AB: CRAC channels and Ca2+ signaling in mast cells. Immunol Rev 2009;231:45–58.
20 Lin LL, Wartmann M, Lin AY, Knopf JL, Seth A, Davis RJ: cPLA2 is phosphorylated and activated by MAP kinase. Cell 1993;72:269–278.
21 Kramer RM, Roberts EF, Um SL, Börsch-Haubold AG, Watson SP, Fisher MJ, Jakubowski JA: p38 mitogen-activated protein kinase phosphorylates cytosolic phospholipaseA2 (cPLA2) in thrombin-stimulated platelets. Evidence that proline-directed phosphorylation is not required for mobilization of arachidonic acid by cPLA2. J Biol Chem 1996;271:27723–27729.
22 Hefner Y, Borsch-Haubold AG, Murakami M, Wilde JI, Pasquet S, Schieltz D, Ghomashchi F, Yates JR 3rd, Armstrong CG, Paterson A, Cohen P, Fukunaga R, Hunter T, Kudo I, Watson SP, Gelb MH: Serine 727 phosphorylation and activation of cytosolic phospholipase A2 by MNK-1-related protein kinases. J Biol Chem 2000;275:37542–37551.
23 Das S, Rafter JD, Kim KP, Gygi SP, Cho W: Mechanism of group IVA cytosolic phospholipase A(2) activation by phosphorylation. J Biol Chem 2003;278:41431–41442.
24 Saito H, Matsumoto K, Okumura S, Kashiwakura J, Oboki K, Yokoi H, Kambe N, Ohta K, Okayama Y: Gene expression profiling of human mast cell subtypes: an in silico study. Allergol Int 2006;55:173–179.
25 Gillespie E: Effects of S-lactoylglutathione and inhibitors of glyoxalase I on histamine release from human leukocytes. Nature 1979;277:135–137.
26 Nishida K, Yamasaki S, Ito Y, Kabu K, Hattori K, Tezuka T, Nishizumi H, Kitamura D, Goitsuka R, Geha RS, Yamamoto T, Yagi T, Hirano T: FcεRI-mediated mast cell degranulation requires calcium-independent microtubule-dependent translocation of granules to the plasma membrane. J Cell Biol 2005;170:115–126.
27 Miyata N, Gon Y, Nunomura S, Endo D, Yamashita K, Matsumoto K, Hashimoto S, Ra C: Inhibitory effects of parthenolide on antigen-induced microtubule formation and degranulation in mast cells. Int Immunopharmacol 2008;8:874–880.

Original Paper

International Archives of Allergy and Immunology

Int Arch Allergy Immunol 2010;152(suppl 1):32–40
DOI: 10.1159/000312123

Published online: June 4, 2010

Salbutamol Modulates the Balance of Th1 and Th2 Cytokines by Mononuclear Cells from Allergic Asthmatics

Takefumi Yamaguchi[a, b] Tomoyuki Soma[a, b] Yotaro Takaku[a, b] Kazuyuki Nakagome[a, b] Koichi Hagiwara[a] Minoru Kanazawa[a] Makoto Nagata[a, b]

[a]Department of Respiratory Medicine and [b]Allergy Center, Saitama Medical University, Saitama, Japan

Key Words

β_2-Agonists · Asthma · IFN-γ · IL-13 · Mononuclear cells · Salbutamol · Th1/Th2 ratio

Abstract

Background: There is evidence that excessive use of inhalational β_2-agonists induces the deterioration of asthma. Although the exact mechanism of this remains to be elucidated, overuse of β_2-agonists may impair the Th1/Th2 balance in asthmatic airways. The aim of the present study was to evaluate whether salbutamol, a representative inhalational β_2-agonist, modifies the production of Th1- and Th2-type cytokines by mononuclear cells separated from patients with asthma and healthy volunteers. ***Methods:*** Peripheral blood mononuclear cells (PBMCs) obtained from 8 healthy volunteers and 10 patients with mild persistent asthma allergic to house dust mites were treated with either salbutamol or medium alone. PBMCs were then stimulated with either medium alone, house dust mite (*Dermatophagoides farina, Df)* allergen or a combination of ionomycin plus phorbol 12-myristate 13-acetate ester (PMA). Concentrations of IFN-γ, IL-13, TNF-α and RANTES in the cell supernatants were measured using ELISA. ***Results:*** In PBMCs from healthy volunteers, salbutamol did not modify IFN-γ production, but increased the spontaneous production of IL-13. In contrast, salbutamol significantly inhibited the spontaneous and ionomycin- plus PMA-stimulated production of IFN-γ by PBMCs from asthmatics. Salbutamol significantly enhanced both spontaneous and *Df*-induced production of IL-13 by PBMCs from asthmatics. Salbutamol did not modify the production of TNF-α. Finally, salbutamol enhanced the production of RANTES induced by *Df* allergen in asthmatics. ***Conclusions:*** Salbutamol inhibits IFN-γ and enhances IL-13 production by PBMCs from asthmatics. These effects would promote a Th1/Th2 imbalance in the airways and may therefore contribute to the deterioration of asthma.

Introduction

Inhalational β_2-adrenergic receptor agonists are representative and supplemental drugs in the treatment of asthma. They can quickly relieve airflow constriction during an asthma attack. However, there is increasing evidence that regular or excessive use of short-acting β_2-agonists (SABAs) is associated with increased allergen-induced airway hyperresponsiveness [1–6], poor asthma control [7–11] and even increased mortality [7, 11]. Interestingly, although β-blockers are generally contraindicated in asthma, an open-label pilot study demonstrated

KARGER

Fax +41 61 306 12 34
E-Mail karger@karger.ch
www.karger.com

1018–2438/10/1525–0032$26.00/0

Accessible online at:
www.karger.com/iaa

Correspondence to: Dr. Makoto Nagata
Department of Respiratory Medicine and Allergy Center
Saitama Medical University
38 Morohongou, Moroyama-cho, Iruma-gun, Saitama 350-0495 (Japan)
Tel. +81 492 76 1637, Fax +81 492 95 8399, E-Mail favre4mn@saitama-med.ac.jp

that an 8-week treatment with the β-blocker nadolol resulted in a dose-dependent increase in airway hyperresponsiveness to methacholine in mild asthma [12].

Neither long-acting β_2-agonists nor SABAs by themselves inhibit allergic bronchial inflammation in asthmatic airways. For example, those drugs do not modify/increase eosinophils in sputum [13–18], yet they increase eosinophil cationic protein and tryptase in induced sputum [13, 14]. β_2-Agonists also do not modify percentages or numbers of mast cells, and CD4 and CD8 lymphocytes in bronchoalveolar lavage fluids [19, 20] or bronchial biopsy specimens [20].

T helper (Th) cells play key roles in modulating the pathogenesis of asthma. Th2 cells play a crucial role in the development of airway inflammation by producing IL-4, IL-5 and IL-13, while Th1 cells produce IFN-γ. β_2-Agonists have been reported to exert suppressive effects on Th1 cytokines [21, 22]. For example, the SABA terbutaline induced a decrease in IFN-γ production in freshly isolated human monocytes stimulated by lipopolysaccharide (LPS) [22]. In contrast, the effects of β_2-agonists on Th2 cytokine production remain controversial. For example, the long-acting β_2-agonist formoterol suppressed allergen-induced IL-5 and IL-13 production by peripheral blood mononuclear cells (PBMCs) [23], while terbutaline increased IL-4 and IL-5 production of tetanus-stimulated human PBMCs [24]. These results suggest that β_2-agonists may alter the Th1/Th2 imbalance in the airways of asthmatics.

In the present study, we assessed whether salbutamol hemisulfate, a representative and widely used SABA, modifies the production of Th1/Th2 cytokines from PBMCs. We report here that this SABA provides a somewhat inhibitory effect on Th1 and an enhancing effect on Th2 cells, thus raising the possibility that β_2-agonists may promote a shift in the Th1/Th2 balance toward Th2 cytokine production in allergic asthma.

Methods

Reagents

Dextran T500 was obtained from Pharmacia Biotech (Uppsala, Sweden). Hanks' balanced salt solution and fetal bovine serum were obtained from Invitrogen (Grand Island, N.Y., USA) and Biomedicals (Aurora, Ohio, USA), respectively. Ionomycin and phorbol 12-myristate 13-acetate (PMA) were obtained from Sigma (St. Louis, Mo., USA). Salbutamol hemisulfate was obtained from Sigma-Aldrich (St. Louis, Mo., USA). *Dermatophagoides farina (Df)* antigen was a kind gift from Torii Pharmaceutical (Tokyo, Japan). The Cell Counting Kit-8 was obtained from Dojindo (Tokyo, Japan).

Table 1. Clinical characteristics of patients with mild persistent allergic asthma

Case, No.	Age, years	Gender	IgE, IU/ml	Eosinophils, n/mm^3
1	23	F	765	780
2	19	F	235	97
3	50	M	229	960
4	27	F	600	700
5	25	F	281	15
6	48	F	186	1,183
7	34	F	167	1,090
8	31	F	109	600
9	25	F	484	252
10	28	M	228	238

Blood Donors

This study was conducted following approval by the Institutional Review Board of the Saitama Medical University Hospital. Informed consent was obtained from all subjects. Eight normal volunteers and 10 patients with allergic asthma with high serum levels of *Df*-specific IgE were enrolled in this study. Normal volunteers consisted of 2 males and 6 females, and ranged in age from 21 to 32 years (mean ± SEM: 26.0 ±1.0 years). The entry criteria for patients with asthma, who met the criteria for mild persistent (step 2) asthma according to the guidelines of the Global Initiative for Asthma published in 2002 [25], were as follows: all patients had previously been treated with inhaled corticosteroid 200–400 μg equivalent to chlorofluorocarbon beclomethasone and had not used oral corticosteroids within 4 weeks prior to study entry; they were nonsmokers and stable for >6 months. Table 1 shows the characteristics of the asthma patients: 2 males and 8 females, ranging in age from 23 to 50 years (mean ± SEM: 32 ± 3), mean IgE was 328 ± 68 IU/ml, and blood eosinophil count was 592 ± 133/mm^3.

Mononuclear Cells

PBMCs were obtained from 40 ml heparinized blood. PBMCs were isolated by the Ficoll-Hypaque density gradient technique and adjusted to a final concentration of 2×10^6 cells/ml in RPMI culture medium (RPMI-1640 supplemented with 10% heat-inactivated fetal calf serum, 100 U/ml penicillin, 100 μg/ml streptomycin and 2 mM L-glutamine). To assess the effects of the drugs, PBMCs were incubated in the presence or absence of 0.1–1 μM salbutamol for 24 h. Subsequently, PBMCs of both normal volunteers and asthma patients were cultured for 72 h at 37°C in 5% CO_2 in the presence or absence of a combination of ionomycin (300 nM, Sigma) and PMA (5 nM, Sigma), or 1 μg/ml *Df* antigen (asthma patients only) [26, 27]. The purity of lymphocytes was >90% in all experiments. The supernatants were stored at –80°C until use.

Measurement of Cytokines and Chemokines

The concentrations of IFN-γ, IL-13, TNF-α and RANTES (regulated upon activation, normal T cell expressed and secreted) in the culture supernatants of PBMCs were measured using ELISA (R&D Systems, Minneapolis, Minn., USA).

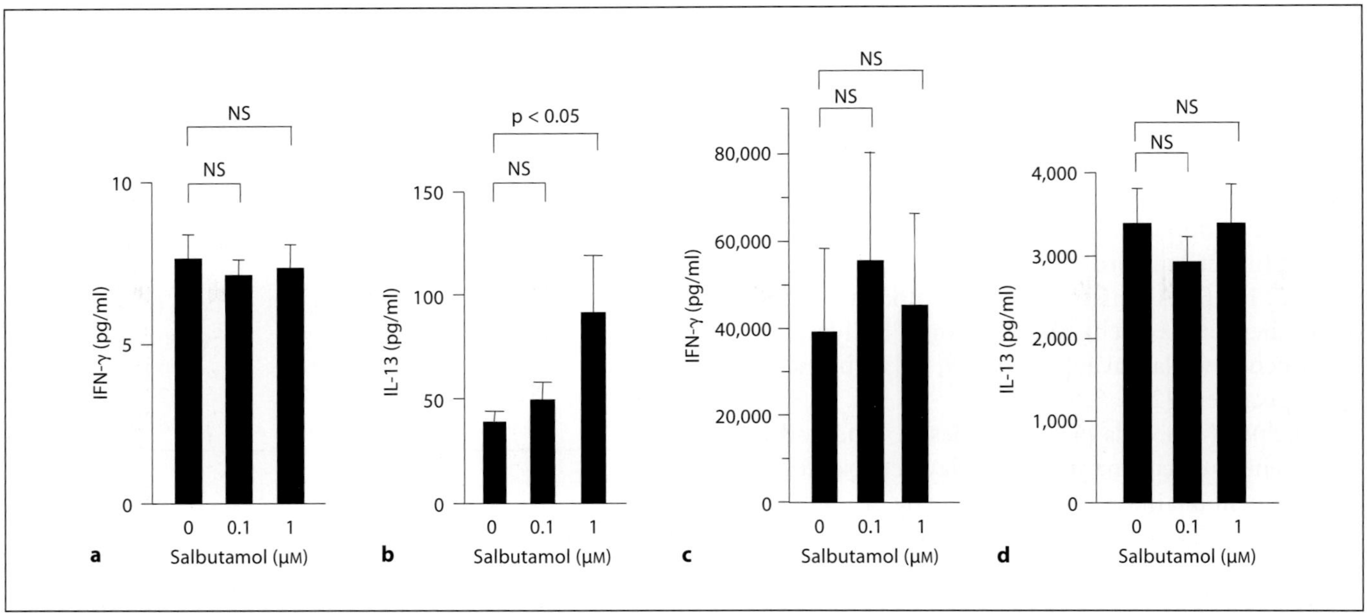

Fig. 1. Effects of salbutamol (0.1 or 1 μM) on the spontaneous production of IFN-γ (**a**) and IL-13 (**b**) by PBMCS of healthy volunteers. Effects of salbutamol (0.1 or 1 μM) on the production of IFN-γ (**c**) and IL-13 (**d**) induced by ionomycin and PMA from PBMCs of healthy volunteers. Means ± SEM from 8 experiments.

Statistical Analysis

Data are presented as means (SEM when variables exhibited normal distribution) or as medians (interquartile ranges when they exhibited abnormal distribution). Student's t test and the Mann-Whitney U test were conducted to compare variables with normal and abnormal distribution, respectively. Non-paired t test was conducted when values were compared between healthy volunteers and patients with allergic asthma. $p < 0.05$ was considered statistically significant.

Results

Salbutamol Enhanced Spontaneous Production of IL-13 by PBMCs from Healthy Volunteers

In the first series of experiments, we assessed the possible effects of salbutamol on IFN-γ and IL-13 production by PBMCs obtained from healthy volunteers. The concentration of IFN-γ from PBMCs was not significantly modified by salbutamol without any stimulation (control: 7.5 ± 0.9 pg/ml; 0.1 μM salbutamol: 7.0 ± 0.6 pg/ml, nonsignificant, NS, vs. control; 1 μM salbutamol: 7.3 ± 0.8 pg/ml, p = NS vs. control, n = 8; fig. 1a). In contrast, the concentration of IL-13 from PBMCs cultured with 1 μM salbutamol (90.9 ± 27.6 pg/ml) was significantly increased compared to control cells without any stimulation (38.9 ± 4.9 pg/ml), with no significant difference between control cells and cells treated with 0.1 μM salbutamol (48.9 ± 8.9 pg/ml; n = 8; fig. 1b). To evaluate whether salbutamol modifies the concentration of IFN-γ or IL-13 in response to a combination of ionomycin and PMA, the supernatants were diluted and concentrations were re-assayed in order that the IFN-γ concentrations were within the detection limits of the assay (1 pg/ml – 10 ng/ml). Neither the IFN-γ (control: 39,587.3 ± 19,002.6 pg/ml; 0.1 μM salbutamol: 55,408.1 ± 25,034.6 pg/ml, 1 μM salbutamol: 45,167.5 ± 20,877.6 pg/ml, p = NS vs. control, respectively; n = 8, fig. 1c) nor the IL-13 concentrations (control: 3,358.9 ± 450.6 pg/ml; 0.1 μM salbutamol: 2,899.0 ± 354.6 pg/ml; 1 μM salbutamol: 3,361.8 ± 500.3 pg/ml, p = NS vs. control, respectively; n = 8, fig. 1d) from PBMCs were modified by salbutamol when the cells were stimulated with 300 nM ionomycin and 5 nM PMA . The total number of viable PBMCs was not significantly modified by 1 μM salbutamol after stimulation with ionomycin and PMA (data not shown) using Cell Counting Kit-8, which is employed to determine viable cell numbers.

Salbutamol Modified IFN-γ and IL-13 Production by PBMCs from Allergic Asthmatics Sensitive to House Dust Mites

We next examined the effect of salbutamol on IFN-γ and IL-13 production by PBMCs obtained from patients

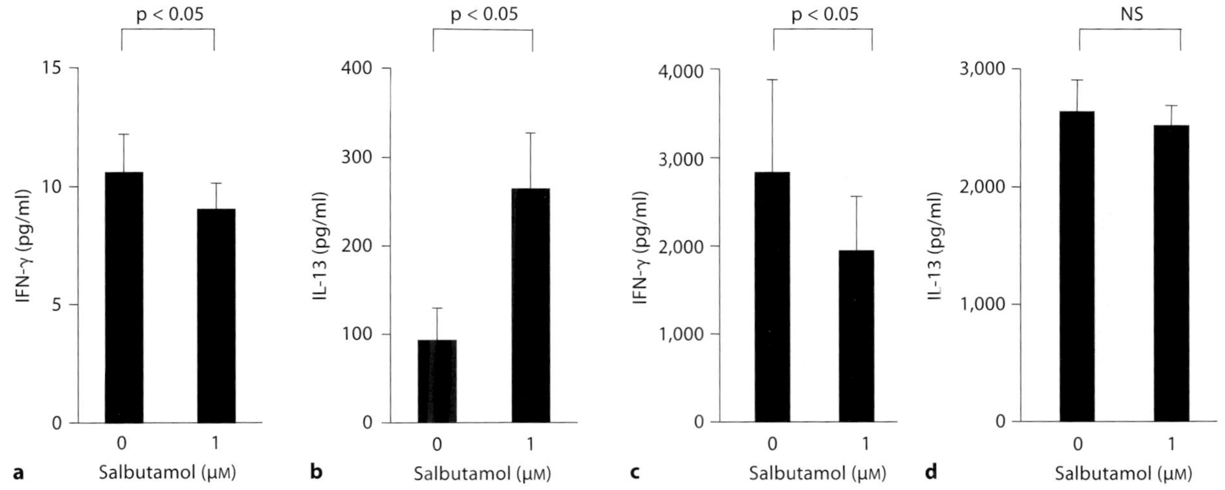

Fig. 2. Effects of salbutamol (1 μM) on the spontaneous production of IFN-γ (**a**) and IL-13 (**b**) by PBMCs of mild persistent asthmatics. Effects of salbutamol (1 μM) on the production of IFN-γ (**c**) and IL-13 (**d**) by PBMCs of mild persistent asthmatics stimulated with ionomycin plus PMA. Means ± SEM from 10 experiments.

with allergic asthma. In this specific series of experiments, activators used to stimulate PBMCs were medium control, 1 μg/ml *Df* antigen, and a combination of ionomycin (300 nM) and PMA (5 nM). Based on the results from healthy donors and because of the limitation of cell numbers, the only salbutamol concentration tested was 1 μM.

Salbutamol significantly reduced the concentration of IFN-γ produced by PBMCs from asthma patients compared to control cells without any stimulation (control: 10.6 ± 1.6 pg/ml; salbutamol: 9.0 ± 1.1 pg/ml, $p < 0.05$, n = 10; fig. 2a). In contrast, salbutamol significantly increased the concentration of IL-13 produced by PBMCs from asthmatics without any stimulation (control: 91.8 ± 37.5 pg/ml; salbutamol: 263.2 ± 63.5 pg/ml, p = 0.04; fig. 2b). When the cells were stimulated with ionomycin and PMA, the baseline concentration of IFN-γ was lower in this population compared with healthy subjects: 39,587.3 ± 19,002.6 (healthy subjects) versus 2,827.1 ± 1,051.6 pg/ml (asthmatics, $p < 0.05$). Salbutamol significantly reduced the concentration of IFN-γ by PBMCs (salbutamol: 1,938.5 ± 630.6 pg/ml, p = 0.03 vs. no drug, n = 10; fig. 2c). IL-13 production induced by ionomycin and PMA was not significantly modified by salbutamol (control: 2,633.7 ± 270.8 pg/ml; salbutamol: 2,515.1 ± 190.5 pg/ml, p = NS, n = 10; fig. 2d). Finally, when PBMCs were stimulated by a specific allergen, namely *Df* antigen, salbutamol did not affect the IFN-γ concentration (control: 12.1 ± 1.5 pg/ml; salbutamol: 10.7 ± 1.2 pg/ml, p = NS, n = 10; fig. 3a); however, the drug significantly enhanced the concentration of IL-13 from PBMCs obtained from allergic asthmatics (control: 126.1 ± 49.3 pg/ml; salbutamol: 292.0 ± 66.8 pg/ml, p = 0.01, n = 10; fig. 3b).

In cells obtained from allergic asthmatics, we next evaluated possible effects of salbutamol on the production of TNF-α, which is capable of enhancing the expression of intercellular adhesion molecule-1 and the production of CXC chemokines (such as IL-8) from endothelial cells, and RANTES (CCL5), which is a CC chemokine capable of eosinophil chemotactic response. Salbutamol did not modify the concentration of TNF-α (control: 38.7 ± 25.0 pg/ml; salbutamol: 31.8 ± 20.9 pg/ml, p = NS, n = 10) and RANTES without any stimulation (control: 424.1 ± 115.7 pg/ml; salbutamol: 520.9 ± 151.6 pg/ml, p = NS, n = 8). However, *Df* allergen was an activator: whereas salbutamol did not modify the concentration of TNF-α (control: 50.9 ± 38.9 pg/ml; salbutamol: 62.7 ± 38.9 pg/ml, p = NS, n = 10; fig. 3c), salbutamol significantly enhanced the concentration of RANTES from PBMCs compared with control (control: 620.2 ± 207.3 pg/ml; salbutamol: 689.4 ± 212.9 pg/ml , $p < 0.05$; fig. 3d).

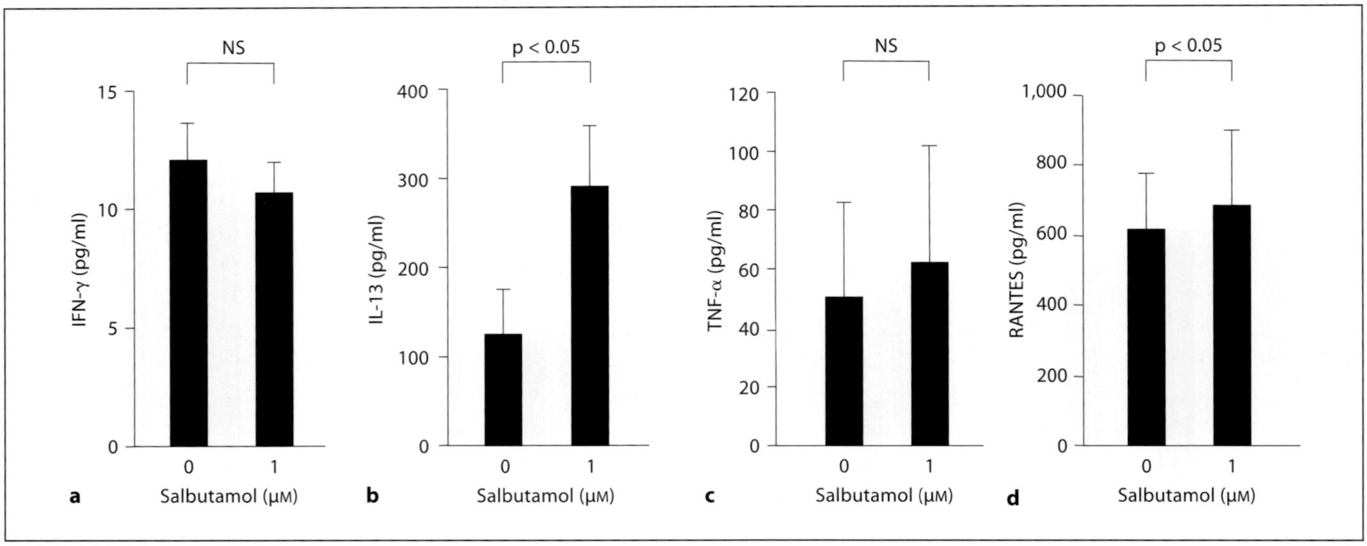

Fig. 3. Effects of salbutamol (1 μM) on the production of IFN-γ (**a**), IL-13 (**b**), TNF-α (**c**) and RANTES (**d**) by PBMCs from mild persistent asthmatics. Means ± SEM from 10 experiments (except for RANTES: 8 experiments).

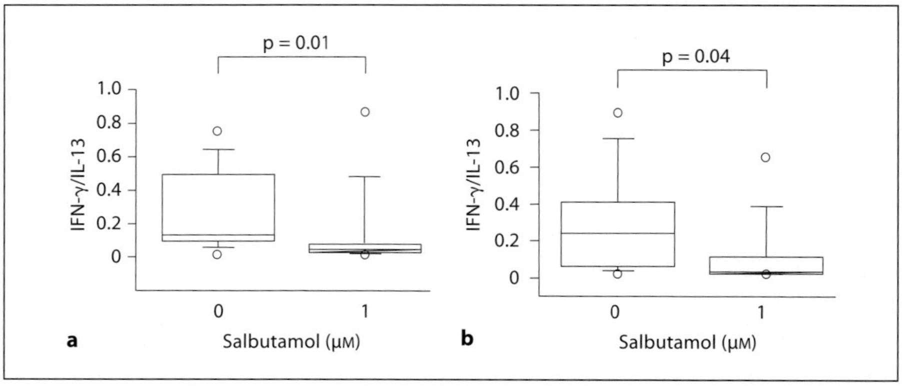

Fig. 4. Salbutamol significantly decreased the ratios of both spontaneous (**a**) and *Df*-allergen-stimulated (**b**) production of IFN-γ/IL-13 in asthmatic donors compared to medium alone [spontaneous production: 0.13 (0.10–0.49) by medium alone and 0.04 (0.02–0.07) by salbutamol, p = 0.01; *Df*-allergen-stimulated production: 0.24 (0.06–0.41) by medium alone and 0.03 (0.02–0.11) by salbutamol, p = 0.04]. Medians (interquartile ranges) from 10 experiments.

Salbutamol Altered the IFN-γ/IL-13 Ratio in Mild Persistent Atopic Asthma

As noted, salbutamol down-modulated IFN-γ and up-regulated IL-13 production under some experimental conditions, raising the possibility that this drug modifies and possibly promotes a shift in the Th1/Th2 balance toward the Th2 phenotype. To confirm this possibility, we calculated the IFN-γ/ IL-13 ratio released by PBMC in the presence or absence of salbutamol. In normal volunteers, salbutamol did not modify the IFN-γ/IL-13 ratio regardless of activators (data not shown). Similarly, salbutamol did not modify the IFN-γ/IL-13 ratio in asthmatic donors when a combination of ionomycin and PMA was the activator (data not shown). On the other hand, 1 μM salbutamol significantly decreased the ratios of both spontaneous and *Df* allergen-stimulated IFN-γ/IL-13 production in asthmatic donors compared with corresponding medium controls (p = 0.01 for spontaneous production, p = 0.04 for *Df* allergen-stimulated production; fig. 4), suggesting that salbutamol leads to a shift in the Th1/Th2 balance toward a Th2-dominant phenotype.

Discussion

In this study, we evaluated the effects of salbutamol, a representative inhalational β_2-agonist, on the production of Th1/Th2 cytokines. First, salbutamol enhanced the spontaneous production of IL-13 by mononuclear cells from healthy volunteers suggesting that salbutamol may act as a stimulator for the generation of this specific Th2 phenotype cytokine. Second, in allergic asthma, salbutamol enhanced both the spontaneous and allergen-specific production of IL-13, while reducing both the spontaneous and ionomycin- plus PMA-stimulated production of IFN-γ. Finally, we observed that salbutamol modestly enhanced the allergen-induced production of RANTES by mononuclear cells of allergic asthmatics. Collectively, these results further suggest that inhalational β_2-agonists such as salbutamol down-modulate the Th1 cytokine response and augment the Th2 cytokine response, and may enhance a shift in the Th1/Th2 balance toward the Th2 phenotype, thus contributing to airway inflammation in asthma.

The reduction in IFN-γ production by salbutamol is consistent with earlier studies about the suppressive effect of β_2-agonists on IFN-γ production. For example, salbutamol has been shown to suppress the production of IL-12, a critical factor driving the development of Th1 cells, by freshly isolated human monocytes stimulated by LPS [28]. Terbutaline also reduced IL-12 production by LPS-stimulated PBMCs and thereby induced a decrease in IFN-γ and increase in IL-4 and IL-5 [24]. These articles suggest that the β_2-agonists are capable of inducing alterations in the Th1/Th2 cytokine balance, at least in part, via a decrease in IL-12 [24]. Additionally, Mizunoa et al. [22] reported that salbutamol and terbutaline inhibit the production of LPS-induced IL-18, an IFN-γ-inducing factor, from monocytes. Moreover, fenoterol inhibits IFN-γ mRNA expression in activated PBMCs obtained from atopic asthmatics, both before and after allergen inhalation challenge [29]. Salbutamol and fenoterol reduce IFN-γ production by normal human PBMCs when stimulated with phytohemagglutinin (PHA) plus PMA for 72 h [30]. Salmeterol and salbutamol (10^{-9}–10^{-5} M) dose-dependently inhibited PHA-induced IFN-γ production by PBMCs from normal volunteers [27]. Formoterol also suppressed *Df* allergen-induced IFN-γ production of PBMCs in a dose-dependent manner [23]. Isoproterenol down-regulates IFN-γ mRNA expression of either concanavalin A (ConA)-stimulated or CD3-activated PBMCs [31] and inhibits IFN-γ production of PMA-stimulated peripheral blood lymphocytes (PBLs) [32].

The effect of salbutamol on IFN-γ production is likely associated with cyclic-AMP (cAMP)-dependent protein kinase A (PKA) activation. β_2-Agonists promote activation of PKA through cAMP elevation [33]. The cAMP-dependent PKA pathway can inhibit the production of cytokines, which may be related to the inhibition of CD3-mediated signaling at its most upstream events by inhibiting activation of $p56^{lck}$ [32]. Other signaling elements that suppress IFN-γ production may include p38 MAPK, in which PMA-stimulated phosphorylation is inhibited by isoproterenol [32]. Isoproterenol also induces attenuation of IFN-γ mRNA expression in ConA-stimulated PBMCs by up-regulating the intracellular cAMP concentration which is blocked by the β_2-adrenal receptor-selective antagonist ICI 118,5511 [31]. In this study, similar signaling pathways may cause inhibition of IFN-γ production. The lack of an inhibitory effect of salbutamol on PMA- or *Df*-induced IFN-γ production may be due to a higher degree of cell activation, different cell populations or different stimulation protocols tested. For example, the stimulation parameters (5 nM PMA for 72 h) in our study are higher and longer than those used in the study by Loza et al. [32], where Th1 and Th2 cytokine induction following a 5-hour treatment of 2 nM PMA was affected by a β-agonist. Changes in the total PBMC number after PMA stimulation in this study, however, suggested that proliferation and viability of PBMCs do not influence IFN-γ production in normal volunteers. Similarly, differences in the salbutamol-induced IFN-γ production between healthy controls and asthmatic donors may at least in part be due to the amount of this cytokine produced: as noted, asthmatics demonstrated a weaker production of IFN-γ.

The exact mechanism by which salbutamol augments IL-13 production remains to be elucidated; however, at a relatively high concentration, β_2-agonists can induce phosphorylation of cAMP response element binding protein (CREB), cAMP downstream effector, following activation of PKA [35, 36]. Phosphorylated CREB interacts with CREB-binding protein in the nucleus, which regulates gene transcription [37]. CREB-binding protein and p300, a nuclear protein, have the ability to regulate the transcription of genes that encode molecules such as IL-4 [38]. The IL-4 gene lies in an area within 140 kb of the IL-13 and IL-5 genes in Th2 lymphocytes [39]. Several intergenic regions of the human IL-4/IL-13 locus have been shown to be transcribed in CD4+ T cells [40]. In Th2 cells, IL-4/IL-13 intergenic transcription is selectively expressed and up-regulated [41]. Collectively, these reports and our results suggest that salbutamol can induce CREB phosphorylation and thereby promote IL-13 gene transcription. Additionally, in this investigation, salbutamol enhanced spontaneous production of IL-13, while reducing IFN-γ, in allergic asthmatics. IFN-γ has broad immune regulatory functions, including suppression of IL-4, IL-5 and IL-13 production [42, 43]. Thus, a reduction in IFN-γ by itself may also partly contribute to enhanced IL-13 production.

Earlier reports about the effects of β_2-agonists on the production of Th2 cytokines and CC chemokines, including IL-13 and RANTES, provide conflicting results. For example, at low concentrations, isoproterenol enhances IL-13 production of PBLs stimulated by CD3 and CD28 [32]. Fenoterol accelerates IL-13 mRNA expression of activated PBMCs obtained from atopic asthmatics after allergen inhalation challenge [29]. Our results concur with these reports in that salbutamol has enhancing effect(s) on Th2 cell cytokine production. The production of other Th2 cytokines was shown to be similarly altered by β-agonists. Terbutaline increased IL-4 and IL-5 production of tetanus-stimulated human PBMCs [24]. Salbutamol and fenoterol failed to decrease IL-4 production by normal human PBMCs when stimulated with PHA and PMA for 72 h [30]. Salmeterol and salbutamol at concentrations $>10^{-9}$ M (up to 10^{-5} M) diminished the inhibitory influence on PHA-induced IL-4 production by PBMCs from normal volunteers [27]. On the other hand, formoterol suppressed allergen-induced IL-5 and IL-13 production of PBMCs in a dose-dependent manner [23]. At high concentrations, isoproterenol directly reduced IL-13 production by CD3-/CD28-stimulated PBLs [32]. Fenoterol inhibited IL-13 mRNA expression in activated PBMC obtained from atopic asthmatics before allergen inhalation challenge [29]. In these studies, experimental conditions varied, including freshly isolated PBLs obtained from health volunteers [33], PBMCs stimulated with 10 μg/ml *Df* allergen (a higher concentration than ours) [23], or stimulation via CD3 and CD28 mAb [29, 32]. The discrepancy in these reports might be due to the different cell populations employed or the different stimulation protocols. Our experimental design includes cytokine generation by cells obtained from patients with allergic asthma in response to relatively low concentrations of a specific allergen, and may therefore closely mimic the clinical situation observed in asthmatics. Moreover, our observation that salbutamol decreased the IFN-γ/IL-13 production in PBLs of patients with allergic asthma suggests that overuse of inhalational β_2-agonists would promote the Th1/Th2 imbalance associated with allergic inflammation of the airways in asthma.

It is unclear whether the cytokine concentrations in supernatant properly represent their production by PBMCs, including synthesis or secretion, because intracellular cytokine concentration was not assessed in our study. The study by Loza et al. [32], which showed that β-agonists modulated the intracellular IFN-γ and IL-13 production by PBLs, allows us to believe that the cytokine concentrations in supernatant represent the new production by PBMCs, although these results need confirmation by future studies. Our experimental condition is closer to the clinical situation than studies in freshly isolated PBLs, T-cell lines or T-cell clones due to the PBMCs employed. Therefore, our results may more closely reflect trafficking of cytokines in the clinical situation.

In our study, salbutamol modestly, but significantly, enhanced RANTES production of PBMCs from allergic asthmatic patients induced by *Df* antigen. This result is consistent with a previous study which reported that formoterol enhanced the expression of macrophage-derived and T-helper cell type 2-related chemokines in human monocytes activated by LPS [44]. RANTES is a representative CC chemokine that promotes recruitment of inflammatory cells, including eosinophils, to allergic inflammation sites, such as bronchial tissue in asthma. Therefore, it is noteworthy that high concentrations of inhalational β_2-agonists in the airways of asthmatics may enhance allergic inflammation through an augmented production of this specific chemokine.

In conclusion, this investigation confirms that the representative inhalational β_2-adrenergic agonist salbutamol induces a shift in the Th1/Th2 cytokine balance toward a Th2 response. This modifying impact is extremely pronounced in cells of allergic asthmatics. Salbutamol also increases RANTES production, which may result in escalated chemotactic behavior of inflammatory cells such as eosinophils. Collectively, high concentrations of inhalational β_2-adrenergic agonists at the bronchial tissue may aggravate allergic inflammation. The exact β_2-agonist concentration in the airways of human asthmatics remains unknown; however, the concentration of these inhalational drugs may be increased in the airways of asthmatic patients who frequently use these drugs due to the lack of exact knowledge of them, severe disease or exacerbation. Such an alteration in cytokine response may, in part, contribute to the exacerbation of asthma in patients frequently taking inhalational β_2-agonists. It is important to note that inhalational β_2-agonists could possibly contribute to the progression of allergic inflammation. Further studies on another β_2-agonists and specific clinical trials are required in the near future.

Disclosure Statement

The authors declare that no financial or other conflict of interest exists in relation to the content of this article.

References

1 Cockcroft DW, McParland CP, Britto SA, Swystun VA, Rutherford BC: Regular inhaled salbutamol and airway responsiveness to allergen. Lancet 1993;342:833–837.

2 Gauvreau GM, Jordana M, Watson RM, Cockroft DW, O'Byrne PM: Effect of regular inhaled albuterol on allergen-induced late responses and sputum eosinophils in asthmatic subjects. Am J Respir Crit Care Med 1997;156:1738–1745.

3 Swystun VA, Gordon JR, Davis EB, Zhang X, Cockcroft DW: Mast cell tryptase release and asthmatic responses to allergen increase with regular use of salbutamol. J Allergy Clin Immunol 2000;106:57–64.

4 Cockcroft DW, O'Byrne PM, Swystun VA, Bhagat R: Regular use of inhaled albuterol and the allergen-induced late asthmatic response. J Allergy Clin Immunol 1995;96:44–49.

5 Lai CK, Twentyman OP, Holgate ST: The effect of an increase in inhaled allergen dose after rimiterol hydrobromide on the occurrence and magnitude of the late asthmatic response and the associated change in nonspecific bronchial responsiveness. Am Rev Respir Dis 1989;140:917–923.

6 Taylor DR, Hannah D: Management of beta-agonist overuse: why and how? J Allergy Clin Immunol 2008;122:836–838.

7 Spitzer WO, Suissa S, Ernst P, Horwitz RI, Habbick B, Cockcroft D, Boivin JF, McNutt M, Buist AS, Rebuck AS: The use of β-agonists and the risk of death and near-death from asthma. N Engl J Med 1992;326:501–506.

8 Drazen JM, Israel E, Boushey HA, Chinchilli VM, Fahy JV, Fish JE, Lazarus SC, Lemanske RF, Martin RJ, Peters SP, Sorkness C, Szefler SJ: Comparison of regularly scheduled with as-needed use of albuterol in mild asthma. Asthma Clinical Research Network. N Engl J Med 1996;335:841–847.

9 Taylor DR, Town GI, Herbison GP, Boothman-Burrell D, Flannery EM, Hancox B, Harré E, Laubscher K, Linscott V, Ramsay CM, Richards G: Asthma control during long-term treatment with regular inhaled salbutamol and salmeterol. Thorax 1998;53:744–752.

10 Lazarus SC, Boushey HA, Fahy JV, Chinchilli VM, Lemanske RF Jr, Sorkness CA, Kraft M, Fish JE, Peters SP, Craig T, Drazen JM, Ford JG, Israel E, Martin RJ, Mauger EA, Nachman SA, Spahn JD, Szefler SJ, Asthma Clinical Research Network for the National Heart, Lung, and Blood Institute: Long-acting β_2-agonist monotherapy vs continued therapy with inhaled corticosteroids in patients with persistent asthma: a randomized controlled trial. JAMA 2001;285:2583–2593.

11 Nelson HS, Weiss ST, Bleecker ER, Yancey SW, Dorinsky PM: SMART Study Group. The salmeterol multicenter asthma research trial: a comparison of usual pharmacotherapy for asthma or usual pharmacotherapy plus salmeterol. Chest 2006;129:15–26.

12 Hanania NA, Singh S, El-Wali R, Flashner M, Franklin AE, Garner WJ, Dickey BF, Parra S, Ruoss S, Shardonofsky F, O'Connor BJ, Page C, Bond RA: The safety and effects of the beta-blocker, nadolol, in mild asthma: an open-label pilot study. Pulm Pharmacol Ther 2008;21:134–141.

13 Turner MO, Johnston PR, Pizzichini E, Pizzichini MM, Hussack PA, Hargreave FE: Anti-inflammatory effects of salmeterol compared with beclomethasone in eosinophilic mild exacerbations of asthma: a randomized, placebo controlled trial. Can Respir J 1998;5:261–268.

14 Aldridge RE, Hancox RJ, Robin Taylor D, Cowan JO, Winn MC, Frampton CM, Town GI: Effects of terbutaline and budesonide on sputum cells and bronchial hyperresponsiveness in asthma. Am J Respir Crit Care Med 2000;161:1459–1464.

15 Manolitsas ND, Wang J, Devalia JL, Trigg CJ, McAulay AE, Davies RJ: Regular albuterol, nedocromil sodium, and bronchial inflammation in asthma. Am J Respir Crit Care Med 1995;151:1925–1930.

16 Swystun VA, Gordon JR, Davis EB, Zhang X, Cockcroft DW: Mast cell tryptase release and asthmatic responses to allergen increase with regular use of salbutamol. J Allergy Clin Immunol 2000;106:57–64.

17 Cockcroft DW, O'Byrne PM, Swystun VA, Bhagat R: Regular use of inhaled albuterol and the allergen-induced late asthmatic response. J Allergy Clin Immunol 1995;96:44–49.

18 Gauvreau GM, Jordana M, Watson RM, Cockroft DW, O'Byrne PM: Effect of regular inhaled albuterol on allergen-induced late responses and sputum eosinophils in asthmatic subjects. Am J Respir Crit Care Med 1997;156:1738–1745.

19 Gardiner PV, Ward C, Booth H, Allison A, Hendrick DJ, Walters EH: Effect of eight weeks of treatment with salmeterol on bronchoalveolar lavage inflammatory indices in asthmatics. Am J Respir Crit Care Med 1994;150:1006–1011.

20 Roberts JA, Bradding P, Britten KM, Walls AF, Wilson S, Gratziou C, Holgate ST, Howarth PH: The long-acting β_2-agonist salmeterol xinafoate: effects on airway inflammation in asthma. Eur Respir J 1999;14:275–282.

21 Panina-Bordignon P, Mazzeo D, Lucia PD, D'Ambrosio D, Lang R, Fabbri L, Self C, Sinigaglia F: β_2-Agonists prevent Th1 development by selective inhibition of interleukin 12. J Clin Invest 1997;100:1513–1519.

22 Mizunoa K, Takahashi HK, Iwagaki H, Katsuno G, Kamurul HASM, Ohtani S, Mori S, Yoshino T, Nishibori M, Tanaka N: β_2-Adrenergic receptor stimulation inhibits LPS-induced IL-18 and IL-12 production in monocytes. Immunol Lett 2005;101:168–172.

23 Hashimoto T, Kitamura N, Kobayashi N, Suko M, Kaminuma O, Mori A: Effect of formoterol on allergen-induced cytokine synthesis by atopic asthmatics. Int Arch Allergy Immunol 2007;143:106–109.

24 Agarwal SK, Marshall GD Jr: Beta-adrenergic modulation of human type-1/type-2 cytokine balance. J Allergy Clin Immunol 2000;105:91–98.

25 Global Initiative for Asthma: Global Strategy for Asthma Management and Prevention. Bethesda, National Institutes of Health, 2002.

26 Nagata M, Shibasaki M, Sakamoto Y, Fukuda T, Makino S, Yamamoto K, Dohi Y: Specific immunotherapy reduces the antigen-dependent production of eosinophil chemotactic activity from mononuclear cells in patients with atopic asthma. J Allergy Clin Immunol 1994;94:160–166.

27 Mohede IC, Van Ark I, Brons FM, Van Oosterhout AJ, Nijkamp FP: Salmeterol inhibits interferon-gamma and interleukin-4 production by human peripheral blood mononuclear cells. Int J Immunopharmacol 1996;18:193–201.

28 Maggi E, Parronchi P, Manetti R, Simonelli C, Piccinni MP, Rugiu FS, De Carli M, Ricci M, Romagnani S: Reciprocal regulatory effects of IFNγ and IL-4 on the in vitro development of human Th1 and Th2 clones. J Immunol 1992;148:2142–2147.

29 Heijink IH, van den Bergez M, Vellengaw E, de Monchy JGR, Postmaz DS, Kauffman HF: Altered β_2-adrenergic regulation of T cell activity after allergen challenge in asthma. Clin Exp Allergy 2004;34:1356–1363.

30 Paul-Eugene N, Kolb JP, Calenda A, Gordon J, Kikutani H, Kishimoto T, Mencia-Huerta JM, Braquet P, Dugas B: Functional interaction between beta 2-adrenoceptor agonists and interleukin-4 in the regulation of CD23 expression and release and IgE production in human. Mol Immunol 1993;30:157–164.

31 Borger P, Hoekstra Y, Esselink MT, Postma DS, Zaagsma J, Vellenga E, Kauffman HF: Beta-adrenoceptor-mediated inhibition of IFN-γ, IL-3, and GM-CSF mRNA accumulation in activated human T lymphocytes is solely mediated by the β_2-adrenoceptor subtype. Am J Respir Cell Mol Biol 1998;19:400–407.

32 Loza MJ, Foster S, Peters SP, Penn RB: Beta-agonists modulate T-cell functions via direct actions on type 1 and type 2 cells. Blood 2006;107:2052–2060.

33 PJ Barnes: Beta-adrenergic receptors and their regulation. Am J Respir Crit Care Med 1995;152:838–860.
34 Ieannin P, Delneste Y, Seveso M, Life P, Bonnefoy JY: IL-12 synergizes with IL-2 and other stimuli in inducing IL-10 production by human T cells. J Immunol 1996;156:3159–3165.
35 Aandahl EM, Moretto WJ, Haslett PA, Vang T, Bryn T, Tasken K, Nixon DF: Inhibition of antigen-specific T cell proliferation and cytokine production by protein kinase A type I. J Immunol 2002;169:802–808.
36 Yamamoto KK, Gonzalez GA, Biggs WH 3rd, Montminy MR: Phosphorylation-induced binding and transcriptional efficacy of nuclear factor CREB. Nature 1988;334:494–498.
37 Chrivia JC, Kwok RP, Lamb N, Hagiwara M, Montminy MR, Goodman RH: Phosphorylated CREB binds specifically to the nuclear protein CBP. Nature 1993;365:855–859.
38 Sisk TJ, Gourley T, Roys S, Chang CH: MHC class II transactivator inhibits IL-4 gene transcription by competing with NF-AT to bind the coactivator CREB binding protein (CBP)/p300. J Immunol 2000;165:2511–2517.
39 Frazer KA, Ueda Y, Zhu Y, Gifford VR, Garofalo MR, Mohandas N, Martin CH, Palazzolo MJ, Cheng JF, Rubin EM: Computational and biological analysis of 680 kb of DNA sequence from the human 5q31 cytokine gene cluster region. Genome Res 1997;7:495.
40 Rogan DF, Cousins DJ, Staynov DZ: Intergenic transcription occurs throughout the human IL-4/IL-13 gene cluster. Biochem Biophys Res Commun 1999;255:556–561.
41 Rogan DF, Cousins DJ, Santangelo S, Ioannou PA, Antoniou M, Lee TH, Staynov DZ: Analysis of intergenic transcription in the human IL-4/IL-13 gene cluster. Proc Natl Acad Sci USA 2004;101:2446–51.
42 Elser B, Lohoff M, Kock S, Giaisi M, Kirchhoff S, Krammer PH, Li-Weber M: IFN-γ represses IL-4 expression via IIRF-1 and IRF-2. Immunity 2002;17:703–712.
43 Nakagome K, Okunishi K, Imamura M, Harada H, Matsumoto T, Tanaka R, Miyazaki J, Yamamoto K, Dohi M: IFN-γ attenuates antigen-induced overall immune response in the airway as a Th1-type immune regulatory cytokine. J Immunol 2009;183:209–220.
44 Hung CH, Chu YT, Hua YM, Hsu SH, Lin CS, Chang HC, Lee MS, Jong YJ: Effects of formoterol and salmeterol on the production of Th1- and Th2-related chemokines by monocytes and bronchial epithelial cells. Eur Respir J 2008;31:1313–1321.

Original Paper

International Archives of Allergy and Immunology

Int Arch Allergy Immunol 2010;152(suppl 1):41–46
DOI: 10.1159/000312124

Published online: June 4, 2010

Changes in Airway Inflammation and Hyperresponsiveness after Inhaled Corticosteroid Cessation in Allergic Asthma

Yotaro Takaku Kazuyuki Nakagome Takehito Kobayashi Takefumi Yamaguchi Fuyumi Nishihara Tomoyuki Soma Koichi Hagiwara Minoru Kanazawa Makoto Nagata

Department of Respiratory Medicine, Allergy Center, Saitama Medical University, Saitama, Japan

Key Words

Airway hyperresponsiveness · Asthma, relapse · *Dermatophagoides farinae* · Eosinophils · House dust mites · Inhaled corticosteroids · Interleukin-4 · Remission, asthma

Abstract

Background: Most patients with asthma are currently controlled by pharmacotherapeutic means such as inhaled corticosteroid (ICS). However, whether ICS actually induces remission of asthma remains unknown. The present study evaluates changes in airway inflammation and hyperresponsiveness in adult patients with asthma after stopping ICS. ***Methods:*** We enrolled 11 patients with allergic asthma (7 males and 4 females; mean age, 52.3 years) who had been asymptomatic and had no exacerbation by low-dose ICS. Airway hyperresponsiveness (AHR) was assessed using methacholine challenge, and induced sputum was evaluated before and every 3 months after ICS cessation during the 1-year follow-up. ***Results:*** Among the 11 asthmatics, AHR increased in 10 (90.9%) and asthma clinically relapsed in 4 (36.4%) within 1 year of ICS cessation. AHR increased in all 7 asthmatics that were sensitized to *Dermatophagoides farinae* and asthma clinically relapsed in 4 (57.1%) of them. Furthermore, eosinophil numbers and IL-4 concentrations in the sputum significantly increased after ICS cessation. ***Conclusions:*** Remission with normal airway response to methacholine (no AHR) might be rare in adult patients with allergic asthma, and sensitization to house dust mites appears to play an important role in relapse. Therefore, ICS cessation should be carefully considered in patients sensitive to house dust mites. Serial determination of eosinophil counts or IL-4 concentrations in sputum might be appropriate for monitoring and preventing asthma relapse in adults.

Introduction

The prevalence of asthma is increasing, and effective pharmacological therapies such as inhaled corticosteroid (ICS) and other management strategies have been developed that have rendered asthma manageable. However, whether ICS could actually induce asthma remission (defined as the absence of asthma symptoms without asthma treatment [1]) was uncertain.

Asthma remission rates are considerably higher in childhood than in adults [2–12]. For example, Vonk et al. [2] reported that 22% of asthmatic children achieved complete remission [defined as the absence of asthma symptoms, no ICS use, normal lung function and no airway hyperresponsiveness (AHR)] and a further 30% achieved clinical remission (no symptoms and no ICS; total 52%) by the age of 32–42 years. In a study by Seker-

KARGER

Fax +41 61 306 12 34
E-Mail karger@karger.ch
www.karger.com

1018–2438/10/1525–0041$26.00/0

Accessible online at:
www.karger.com/iaa

Correspondence to: Dr. Makoto Nagata
Department of Respiratory Medicine and Allergy Center
Saitama Medical University
38 Morohongou, Moroyama-cho, Iruma-gun, Saitama 350-0495 (Japan)
Tel. +81 492 76 1637, Fax +81 492 95 8399, E-Mail favre4mn@saitama-med.ac.jp

el et al. [3], 27% and a further 26% of asthmatic children achieved complete remission (no symptoms, no medications, normal lung function and no AHR) and clinical remission (no symptoms and no medications), respectively, by the age of 17 years. Age at onset [4], disease duration [4], response to initial treatment [2, 5], forced expiratory volume in 1 s (FEV_1) at onset [2, 5–9], AHR at onset [6–9], total IgE [5–11], female gender [3, 6] or sensitization to house dust mites [8, 10] were predictive factors for remission or relapse of childhood asthma.

In contrast, little information is available regarding remission or relapse of adult asthma. Therefore, the prognosis of adult asthma is not understood in detail, and how treatment could be reduced or stopped has not been fully clarified. The Global Initiative for Asthma guidelines recommend that therapies for asthma control, e.g. ICS, can be stopped if asthma remains controlled in patients on the lowest dose and symptoms do not recur for 1 year [12]. However, the guidelines also indicate that little experimental data support the optimal timing, sequence and magnitude of reductions or cessation of treatment for asthmatic adults [12].

The present study investigates whether ICS administration could be stopped in adult asthmatics without relapse or AHR induction. We also evaluated changes in airway inflammation and AHR after ICS cessation.

Patients and Methods

Patients and Study Protocol

This observational study was conducted in the Allergy and Asthma Center of the Saitama Medical University Hospital after receiving approval from the Institutional Review Board of the Hospital and written informed consent from all patients who participated. Adult asthmatics that had been asymptomatic by low-dose ICS (fluticasone propionate 100 μg b.i.d. or equivalent) were evaluated for 12 months after ICS cessation. Asthma was diagnosed based on a history of recurrent wheezing, dyspnea, chest tightness and either reversible airflow limitation (FEV_1 <70% of predicted or a previous best value that increased by >15% after the inhalation of 200 μg salbutamol) or methacholine (MCh)-induced AHR. Before enrolment, we confirmed that the patients had been regularly treated with ICS for at least 6 months without regular long-acting bronchodilators, and that they had been asymptomatic and stable on low-dose ICS over the past 3 months. Eleven adult patients (7 males and 4 females, mean age 52.3 years, range: 30–71 years) participated in the study. All were atopic according to positive skin prick tests or had specific IgE antibody in response to common inhalant allergens such as house dust mites *(Dermatophagoides farinae, Df)*. None of the patients had any other respiratory or systemic disease.

At the start of the run-in period, all of the patients recorded symptom scores and peak expiratory flow rates (PEFR) using a diary. At the end of the run-in period, all of them underwent baseline spirometry, the MCh challenge test and sputum evaluation for inflammation. To proceed to ICS cessation, asthma had to be 'controlled'. We defined 'controlled' asthma based on the definition of 'totally controlled' asthma in the Gaining Optimal Asthma ControL (GOAL) study [13] except for the evaluation of 'morning PEF'. (We used 'over 80% personal best' criteria, but not 'over 80% predicted' criteria [13].) After treatment cessation, all patients underwent the MCh challenge test and sputum evaluation every 3 months, and PEFR was monitored and symptoms were managed for 12 months. Relapse was defined as insufficient asthma control according to the GOAL study [13].

Monitoring PEFR and Asthmatic Symptoms

All of the patients monitored PEFR using a mini-Wright Peak Flow Meter twice daily (early morning and at bedtime before drug inhalation) for 3 consecutive months at the start of the study (run-in period) and then for up to 12 months. The weekly mean of the highest value of three exhalations into the meter (mean PEFR) was recorded in their diaries and evaluated. All patients also recorded asthmatic symptoms (cough, dyspnea and wheezing) in their diaries.

Pulmonary Function and MCh Challenge Tests

Pulmonary function tests were performed according to the American Thoracic Society guidelines [14] using an AS307 spirometer (Minato Medical Science, Osaka, Japan) and the MCh challenge proceeded as described previously [15, 16]. Briefly, baseline FEV_1 was recorded and then, after confirming that FEV_1 did not fall with an inhalation of saline, increasing concentrations of MCh (39–20,000 μg) were delivered using a DeVilbiss 646 jet nebulizer every 2 min, and FEV_1 was measured immediately after each inhalation. The concentration of MCh that induced a 20% fall in FEV_1 was calculated from the semi-log scale dose-response curve and is expressed as PD_{20} FEV_1 (cumulative dose producing a 20% fall in FEV_1).

Sputum Induction and Processing

Sputum was induced as described previously [17–19]. Salbutamol was delivered using a metered dose inhaler. Fifteen minutes later, sterile hypertonic saline (4.5%) was inhaled using an ultrasonic nebulizer at room temperature. Sputum was collected at 5-min intervals for up to 30 min. Rinsing with mouthwash before each expectoration was encouraged to minimize salivary contamination. All initial samples were discarded. Induced sputum samples collected into 50-ml polypropylene tubes were stored at 4°C for processing. Hanks' balanced salt solution (HBSS; 1 ml) containing 1% dithiothreitol (Sigma, St. Louis, Mo., USA) was added to sputum samples, which were then vortex mixed and repeatedly aspirated at ambient temperature until the mixture was homogeneous. Samples were diluted with HBSS to 5 ml, and separated by centrifugation at 400 *g* for 10 min. Cytokine concentrations were measured in supernatants, and cytospin slides of resuspended pellets were stained with May-Giemsa for differential cell counts. At least 500 inflammatory cells were counted for each sample. Cytospin slides were judged as adequate when <50% of squamous epithelial cells were present. Concentrations of IFN-γ and IL-4 in sputum supernatants were measured using Bio-Plex assay kits (Bio-Rad, Mississauga, Ont., Canada).

Table 1. Clinical characteristics of the patients

Patients No.	sex	age years	Disease duration years	FEV_1 % of predicted	Total IgE IU/ml	Specific IgE Ab to mite	Pets	Pediatric asthma	Smoking
1	F	67	7	105	33	–	dog	–	–
2	M	60	14	91	73	–	–	–	–
3	M	71	15	66	985	–	cat	–	–
4	F	64	17	89	188	+	cat	–	–
5	M	34	31	66	364	+	–	+	–
6	M	59	14	72	639	+	–	–	+
7	F	44	6	98	396	+	cat	–	–
8	M	30	1	112	524	+	–	–	–
9	M	63	23	72	67	–	cat	–	–
10	M	53	27	85	32	+	–	+	–
11	F	30	10	94	1,443	+	–	–	–

Table 2. Outcome after ICS cessation

Patient No.	PD_{20}, μg/ml before	PD_{20}, μg/ml after	Recurrence
1	>20,000	312	–
2	>20,000	<78	–
3	154	78	–
4	3,375	ND	+ (10)
5	624	ND	+ (4)
6	1,812	ND	+ (16)
7	>20,000	4,750	–
8	>20,000	18,500	–
9	1,125	468	–
10	2,375	ND	+ (12)
11	2,812	1,875	–

ND = Not done. Mean duration of asthma recurrence after ICS is shown in parentheses (in weeks).

Statistical Analysis

Statistical significance was determined using the Kruskal-Wallis test. $p < 0.05$ was considered to indicate a statistically significant difference. Values are shown as means ± SEM.

Results

Treatment with ICS was discontinued in 11 patients with asthma that was 'controlled' by a minimal dose of ICS (fluticasone propionate 100 μg b.i.d. or equivalent) for >3 months. All of them had allergic asthma, 9 had adult-onset and 2 had a history of pediatric asthma. Ten were nonsmokers, 1 currently smoked, and 1 had used a short-acting β_2-agonist within the past year. In 8 patients, the duration of asthma was >10 years and FEV_1 was <70% of predicted in 2 of them (table 1).

Within 1 year of stopping ICS, AHR worsened in 10 (90.9%) of the 11 patients and asthma recurred in 4 (36.4%) of them (table 2). Asthma symptoms recurred in some patients immediately after ICS cessation and in all of them within 4 months. All of those with clinical asthma relapse were sensitized to *Df*, and the 1 current smoker as well as the patient who had used the short-acting β_2-agonist within the past year also relapsed. Of the 7 patients with specific IgE antibody against *Df*, AHR aggravated in all of them and asthma recurred in 4 (57.1%). AHR worsened in all 5 patients with a pet (dog or cat). Four patients without AHR during the run-in period have remained asymptomatic for 1 year (tables 1, 2).

Sputum was obtained from 9 patients. After ICS cessation, AHR worsened in 8 of them and 3 relapsed. The ratio of eosinophils in sputum obtained immediately before asthma relapse or AHR induction was significantly increased compared with that obtained during the run-in period (2.1 ± 0.6 vs. 1.1 ± 0.3%, $p < 0.05$; fig. 1). Macrophages, neutrophils, lymphocytes and total cell counts in sputum did not significantly differ (data not shown).

We measured cytokine concentrations in the sputum from 6 patients. After ICS cessation, AHR worsened in all patients and 2 relapsed. The IFN-γ concentration did not significantly change after ICS cessation (before vs. after cessation: 46.1 ± 10.6 vs. 34.6 ± 6.1 pg/ml; fig. 2). In contrast, the IL-4 concentration in sputum obtained just before asthma relapse or AHR induction was significantly increased compared with that during the run-in period (2.8 ± 0.8 vs. 1.5 ± 0.5 pg/ml, $p < 0.05$; fig. 2).

Among other potential predictors of asthma recurrence, the influence of disease duration, ICS treatment duration, lung function (e.g. FEV_1 and PEFR) or eosinophils in peripheral blood were also investigated, but none was associated with clinical relapse.

Discussion

We demonstrated that among 11 adult patients with allergic asthma 'controlled' by low-dose ICS alone, ICS cessation induced an increase in AHR in 10 (90.9%) of them and asthma relapse in 4 (36.4%). The discontinua-

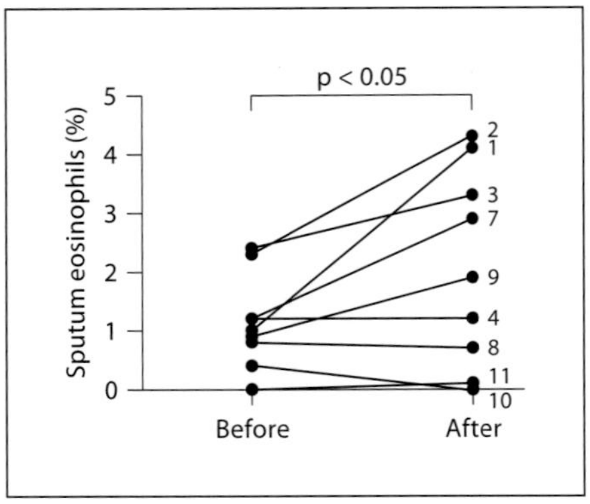

Fig. 1. Changes in sputum eosinophil ratios (%) after ICS cessation. Sputum was obtained from adult asthmatics (n = 9) during the run-in period (before cessation of ICS) or at the end of the study (after ICS cessation). Eosinophils were identified by May-Giemsa staining and morphologically. Patient numbers are shown on the right.

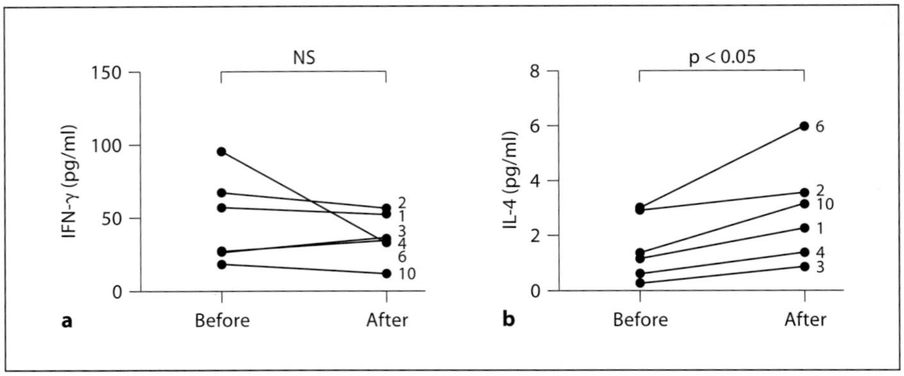

Fig. 2. Changes in IFN-γ (**a**) and IL-4 concentrations (**b**) in sputum after ICS cessation. Sputum was obtained from adult asthmatics (n = 6) during the run-in period (before cessation of ICS) or at the end of the study (after ICS cessation). Concentrations of IFN-γ or IL-4 in sputum supernatant are shown. Patient numbers are shown on the right. NS = Nonsignificant.

tion of ICS resulted in an increase in AHR in all 7 *Df*-sensitized adult asthmatics and asthma relapse in 4 (57.1%). The 4 who clinically relapsed were all sensitized to *Df.* Eosinophil numbers and IL-4 concentrations increased in sputum immediately before asthma relapse or AHR induction. These results indicate that remission in adult patients with allergic asthma, especially among those who are sensitized to house dust mites, is rare. The results also suggest that the eosinophil count or IL-4 concentration in sputum after ICS cessation could be an important predictive factor for relapse in adult asthma.

There is no standardized definition about complete remission or clinical remission in adult asthma. In this study, we used the term 'remission', but not 'complete remission' or 'clinical remission', according to the definition by the Japanese Pediatric Guidelines for the Treatment and Management of Asthma [1], as we evaluated patients only 1 year after ICS cessation. Our results demonstrated that only 1 patient (9.1%) achieved remission with normal airway response to MCh (no AHR) even 1 year after ICS cessation (table 2). Six patients had AHR without asthma symptoms for 1 year (54.5%), and asthma relapsed in 4 (36.4%) patients, all of whom relapsed within 4 months (table 2). Panhuysen et al. [20] studied 181 asthma patients aged 13–44 years at enrolment and found that only 11% remained in remission with no AHR and normal lung function after 25 years. Moreover, recent reports suggest that about 50% of adult asthmatics relapse within 1 year after ICS cessation [21–23], and that most clinical relapses occur within 3 months [21, 24]. Therefore, our results were consistent with these previous studies and confirmed that remission with no AHR in adult asthma would be more difficult to achieve. As increasing evidence indicates that airway inflammation is present during the remission of allergic asthma [25], our results might support the significance of an anti-inflammatory strategy, such as ICS therapy for asymptomatic adult asthmatics, but further studies are required.

AHR worsened in 10 (90.9%) of the 11 patients with allergic asthma after ICS cessation, and asthma recurred in 4 (36.4%) of them (table 2). Of the 7 *Df*-sensitized adult asthmatics, AHR was aggravated in all of them and asthma recurred in 4 (57.1%). Therefore, the atopic status, especially sensitization to house dust mites, may play an important role in the pathogenesis of asthma relapse, leading to the hypothesis that relapse in allergic asthma might be inevitable unless allergen avoidance is completely achieved. In childhood asthma, Bjerg-Bäcklund et al. [26] reported that the frequency of remission was significantly higher in non-allergic asthmatics than in allergic asthmatics. Limb et al. [11] reported that lower IgE levels and fewer positive allergy skin tests in addition to milder symptoms were factors predictive of remission of moderate-severe asthma. Sears et al. [27] reported that factors predictive of relapse were childhood sensitization to house dust mites as well as AHR and early age at onset. Our results in adult asthma were consistent with these findings in childhood asthma. Moreover, sensitization to inhalant allergens, e.g. house dust mites, increases the risk of developing asthma [28, 29]. Toelle et al. [6] demonstrated that in addition to a low FEV_1 and AHR, atopy in childhood is a predictive factor for having asthma in adulthood. In a study by Visser et al. [7] the increase in AHR after ICS withdrawal was associated with more atopic features (positive RAST and high IgE) as well as lower FEV_1 levels, indicating that continued sensitization to house dust mites could trigger the development of asthma or the increase in AHR.

Eosinophils and IL-4 concentrations in sputum increased immediately before asthma relapse or AHR induction (fig. 1, 2), suggesting that the Th2-mediated immune response played an important role in these processes. Eosinophils release various lipid mediators, cytokines and growth factors involved in the pathogenesis of asthma [30]. IL-4 drives B-cell isotype switching from IgM to IgE [31] and augments eosinophil adhesion to and transmigration of eosinophils through the endothelium by enhancing the expression of adhesion molecules on endothelial cells [32], thus initiating eosinophil infiltration into the airways. In a report by Masuyama et al. [33], intranasal corticosteroid inhibited eosinophilic nasal inflammation and mRNA expression of IL-4 in the nasal mucosa, suggesting that IL-4 would mediate the development of eosinophilic inflammation in the airways. In a mouse model of allergic airway inflammation, To et al. [34] reported that antigen systemic sensitization could induce AHR and increase IL-4 concentration in bronchoalveolar lavage fluid before or at the early phase of eosinophilic airway inflammation. Therefore, IL-4 played an essential role in the increase in AHR at the early phase of eosinophilic airway inflammation, which was consistent with our results.

The effect of eosinophil counts in sputum on the prevention of asthma exacerbation has recently been highlighted [35], and Deykin et al. reported that asthma relapse in children is associated with an increased number of eosinophils in sputum [36]. Furthermore, Giannini et al. [23] reported that sputum eosinophil ratios significantly increase during symptom recurrence in adult asthmatics after ICS cessation. Therefore, evaluation of eosinophils in sputum would be a reasonable strategy for monitoring and preventing asthma relapse. Serial measurements of Th2 cytokines such as IL-4 in sputum might also be useful for monitoring.

However, limitations of this study were the small study cohort (only 11 patients participated in this study) and the allergic type of their asthma. Therefore, caution should be applied when extrapolating the findings of this study to all asthmatics. Further studies are required to clarify changes in eosinophil ratios and IL-4 concentrations in sputum after ICS cessation in all types of asthma, including non-allergic asthma.

In conclusion, we demonstrated that remission in adult patients with allergic asthma, especially those who are allergic to house dust mites, is difficult to achieve. Eosinophil ratios and IL-4 concentrations in sputum increased immediately before asthma relapse or AHR induction. Therefore, ICS cessation should be carefully considered in *Df*-sensitized adult asthmatics. Serial examination of eosinophil counts or IL-4 concentrations in sputum might provides a reasonable and useful strategy for monitoring and preventing asthma relapse.

Acknowledgments

We wish to express our gratitude to Ms. Akemi Yokote for her excellent technical assistance. This work was supported by a Health Labor Science Research grant.

Disclosure Statement

The authors declare that no financial or other conflict of interest exists in relation to the content of this article.

References

1 Japanese Society of Allergy and Clinical Immunology: Japanese Pediatric Guidelines for the Treatment and Management of Asthma 2008. Tokyo, Kyowa Kikaku, 2008.
2 Vonk JM, Postma DS, Boezen HM, Grol MH, Schouten JP, Koëter GH, Gerritsen J: Childhood factors associated with asthma remission after 30 year follow up. Thorax 2004;59: 925–929.
3 Sekerel BE, Civelek E, Karabulut E, Yildirim S, Tuncer A, Adalioglu G: Are risk factors of childhood asthma predicting disease persistence in early adulthood different in the developing world? Allergy 2006;61:869–877.
4 De Marco R, Locatelli F, Cerveri I, Bugiani M, Marinoni A, Giammanco G, Italian Study on Asthma in Young Adults Study Group: Incidence and remission of asthma: a retrospective study on the natural history of asthma in Italy. J Allergy Clin Immunol 2002;110:228–235.

5 Grol MH, Postma DS, Vonk JM, Schouten JP, Rijcken B, Koëter GH, Gerritsen J: Risk factors from childhood to adulthood for bronchial responsiveness at age 32–42 yr. Am J Respir Crit Care Med 1999;160:150–156.
6 Toelle BG, Xuan W, Peat JK, Marks GB: Childhood factors that predict asthma in young adulthood. Eur Respir J 2004;23:66–70.
7 Visser MJ, Brand PL, Boezen HM, van Aalderen WM, Kauffman HF, Postma DS: Clinical and immunologic factors associated with the presence or absence of airways hyper-responsiveness in childhood asthma. Clin Exp Allergy 2002;32:1278–1284.
8 Taylor DR, Cowan JO, Greene JM, Willan AR, Sears MR: Asthma in remission. Can relapse in early adulthood be predicted at 18 years of age? Chest 2005;127:845–850.
9 Nagata S, Ago Y, Teshima H, Imada Y: Atopic disposition and bronchial reactivity to inhaled acetylcholine in young adults with a history of asthma in childhood. J Asthma 1984;21:151–159.
10 Illi S, von Mutius E, Lau S, Nickel R, Niggemann B, Sommerfeld C, Wahn U, Multicenter Allergy Study Group: The pattern of atopic sensitization is associated with the development of asthma in childhood. J Allergy Clin Immunol 2001;108:709–714.
11 Limb SL, Brown KC, Wood RA, Wise RA, Eggleston PA, Tonascia J, Hamilton RG, Adkinson NF Jr: Adult asthma severity in individuals with a history of childhood asthma. J Allergy Clin Immunol 2005;115:61–66.
12 Global Initiative for Asthma: Global Strategy for Asthma Management and Prevention 2008 (update). Bethesda, National Institutes of Health, 2008.
13 Bateman ED, Boushey HA, Bousquet J, Busse WW, Clark TJ, Pauwels RA, Pedersen SE, GOAL Investigators Group: Can guideline-defined asthma control be achieved? The Gaining Optimal Asthma ControL study. Am J Respir Crit Care Med 2004;170:836–844.
14 American Thoracic Society: Lung function testing: selection of reference values and interpretative strategies. Am Rev Respir Dis 1991;144:1202–1218.
15 Chai H, Farr RS, Froehlich LA, Mathison DA, McLean JA, Rosenthal RR, Sheffer AL, Spector SL, Townley RG: Standardization of bronchial inhalation challenge procedures. J Allergy Clin Immunol 1975;56:323–327.
16 Paggiaro PL, Dente FL, Morelli MC, Bancalari L, Di Franco A, Giannini D, Vagaggini B, Bacci E, Fabbri LM, Giuntini C: Postallergen inhaled budesonide reduces late asthmatic response and inhibits the associated increase of airway responsiveness to methacholine in asthmatics. Am J Respir Crit Care Med 1994; 149:1447–1451.
17 Keatings VM, Evans DJ, O'Connor BJ, Barnes PJ: Cellular profiles in asthmatic airways: a comparison of induced sputum, bronchial washings, and bronchoalveolar lavage fluid. Thorax 1997;52:372–374.
18 Bacci E, Cianchetti S, Paggiaro PL, Carnevali S, Bancalari L, Dente FL, Di Franco A, Giannini D, Vagaggini B, Giuntini C: Comparison between hypertonic and isotonic saline-induced sputum in the evaluation of airway inflammation in subjects with moderate asthma. Clin Exp Allergy 1996;26: 1395–1400.
19 Paggiaro PL, Chanez P, Holz O, Ind PW, Djukanovic R, Maestrelli P, Sterk PJ: Sputum induction. Eur Respir J 2002;37:3s–8s.
20 Panhuysen CI, Vonk JM, Koëter GH, Schouten JP, van Altena R, Bleecker ER, Postma DS: Adult patients may outgrow their asthma: a 25-year follow-up study. Am J Respir Crit Care Med 1997;155:1267–1272.
21 Haahtela T, Järvinen M, Kava T, Kiviranta K, Koskinen S, Lehtonen K, Nikander K, Persson T, Selroos O, Sovijärvi A, Stenius-Aarniala B, Svahn T, Tammivaara R, Laitinen LA: Effects of reducing or discontinuing inhaled budesonide in patients with mild asthma. N Engl J Med 1994;331:700–705.
22 Marabini A, Cardinalini G, Severini C, Ripandelli A, Siracusa A: Is normal bronchial responsiveness in asthmatics a reliable index for withdrawing inhaled corticosteroid treatment? Chest 1998;113:964–967.
23 Giannini D, Di Franco A, Cianchetti S, Bacci E, Dente FL, Vagaggini B, Paggiaro PL: Analysis of induced sputum before and after withdrawal or treatment with inhaled corticosteroids in asthmatic patients. Clin Exp Allergy 2000;30:1777–1784.
24 Waalkens HJ, Van Essen-Zandvliet EE, Hughes MD, Gerritsen J, Duiverman EJ, Knol K, Kerrebijn KF: Cessation of long-term treatment with inhaled corticosteroid (budesonide) in children with asthma results in deterioration. The Dutch CNSLD Study Group. Am Rev Respir Dis 1993;148:1252–1257.
25 van den Toorn LM, Overbeek SE, de Jongste JC, Leman K, Hoogsteden HC, Prins JB: Airway inflammation is present during clinical remission of atopic asthma. Am J Respir Crit Care Med 2001;164:2107–2113.
26 Bjerg-Bäcklund A, Perzanowski MS, Platts-Mills T, Sandström T, Lundbäck B, Rönmark E: Asthma during the primary school ages – prevalence, remission and the impact of allergic sensitization. Allergy 2006;61: 549–555.
27 Sears MR, Greene JM, Willan AR, Wiecek EM, Taylor DR, Flannery EM, Cowan JO, Herbison GP, Silva PA, Poulton R: A longitudinal, population-based, cohort study of childhood asthma followed to adulthood. N Engl J Med 2003;349:1414–1422.
28 Sporik R, Holgate ST, Platts-Mills TA, Cogswell JJ: Exposure to house-dust mite allergen (Der p I) and the development of asthma in childhood. A prospective study. N Engl J Med 1990;323:502–507.
29 de Kluijver J, Evertse CE, Schrumpf JA, van der Veen H, Zwinderman AH, Hiemstra PS, Rabe KF, Sterk PJ: Asymptomatic worsening of airway inflammation during low-dose allergen exposure in asthma: protection by inhaled steroids. Am J Respir Crit Care Med 2002;166:294–300.
30 Gleich GJ: Mechanisms of eosinophil-associated inflammation. J Allergy Clin Immunol 2000;105:651–663.
31 Broide DH: Molecular and cellular mechanisms of allergic disease. J Allergy Clin Immunol 2001;108:S65–S71.
32 Nagata M, Sedgwick JB, Bates ME, Kita H, Busse WW: Eosinophil adhesion to vascular cell adhesion molecule-1 activates superoxide anion generation. J Immunol 1995;155: 2194–2202.
33 Masuyama K, Jacobson MR, Rak S, Meng Q, Sudderick RM, Kay AB, Lowhagen O, Hamid Q, Durham SR: Topical glucocorticosteroid (fluticasone propionate) inhibits cells expressing cytokine mRNA for interleukin-4 in the nasal mucosa in allergen-induced rhinitis. Immunology 1994;82:192–199.
34 To Y, Dohi M, Tanaka R, Sato A, Nakagome K, Yamamoto K: Early interleukin 4-dependent response can induce airway hyperreactivity before development of airway inflammation in a mouse model of asthma. Lab Invest 2001;81:1385–1396.
35 Green RH, Brightling CE, McKenna S, Hargadon B, Parker D, Bradding P, Wardlaw AJ, Pavord ID: Asthma exacerbations and sputum eosinophil counts: a randomised controlled trial. Lancet 2002;360:1715–1721.
36 Deykin A, Lazarus SC, Fahy JV, Wechsler ME, Boushey HA, Chinchilli VM, Craig TJ, Dimango E, Kraft M, Leone F, Lemanske RF, Martin RJ, Pesola GR, Peters SP, Sorkness CA, Szefler SJ, Israel E, Asthma Clinical Research Network, National Heart, Lung, and Blood Institute/NIH: Sputum eosinophil counts predict asthma control after discontinuation of inhaled corticosteroids. J Allergy Clin Immunol 2005;115:720–727.

Original Paper

International Archives of Allergy and Immunology

Int Arch Allergy Immunol 2010;152(suppl 1):47–53
DOI: 10.1159/000312125

Published online: June 4, 2010

Role of Th2 Cells in IgG4-Related Lacrimal Gland Enlargement

Hiroko Kanari[c] Shin-ichiro Kagami[a, c] Daisuke Kashiwakuma[a, c] Yoshihiro Oya[a] Shunsuke Furuta[b] Kei Ikeda[a] Akira Suto[a, c] Kotaro Suzuki[a, c] Koichi Hirose[a] Norihiko Watanabe[a] Yoshitaka Okamoto[d] Shuichi Yamamoto[e] Itsuo Iwamoto[b] Hiroshi Nakajima[a, c]

[a]Department of Allergy and Clinical Immunology, Chiba University Hospital, [b]Research Center for Allergy and Clinical Immunology, Asahi General Hospital, and Departments of [c]Molecular Genetics, [d]Otolaryngology, Head and Neck Surgery, and [e]Ophthalmology and Visual Science, Graduate School of Medicine, Chiba University, Chiba, Japan

Key Words

Asthma · Eosinophils · IgE · IgG4 · Lacrimal gland enlargement

Abstract

Background: Lacrimal gland enlargement (LGE) is one of the characteristics of Mikulicz's disease (MD). Recently, marked serum IgG4 elevation and infiltration of IgG4-positive plasmacytes in the enlarged exocrine glands have been reported in MD patients. However, little is known about the role of CD4+ T cells and their cytokines in IgG4-related diseases. The aim of this study was to evaluate the characteristics of CD4+ T cells in patients with IgG4-related diseases. ***Methods:*** We investigated the clinical characteristics of 9 patients with LGE and elevated serum IgG4 levels (named IgG4-related LGE). We also examined mRNA expression of cytokines and transcription factors of peripheral blood CD4+ T cells in patients with IgG4-related LGE. ***Results:*** All patients with IgG4-related LGE showed elevated serum IgE levels. In addition, 5 of 9 patients with IgG4-related LGE exhibited eosinophilia and asthma-like symptoms. In patients with IgG4-related LGE, mRNA expression of IL-4, IL-5, IL-10 and GATA-3 but not IFN-γ or T-bet was enhanced on CD4+ T cells compared with that in healthy controls. ***Conclusions:*** Th2 cells may be involved in the pathogenesis of IgG4-related diseases.

Introduction

The unique condition characterizing Mikulicz's disease (MD) is the idiopathic and symmetrical enlargement of the lacrimal, submandibular and parotid glands. MD has been considered as a subtype of Sjögren's syndrome (SjS) because Morgan and Castleman [1] have concluded that MD and SjS are the same entity on the basis of histopathological similarity. However, several reports have demonstrated that MD differs from SjS with respect to some clinical features and laboratory findings [2–4]: e.g. MD patients lack anti-SS-A and anti-SS-B antibodies, whereas SjS patients frequently have these antibodies. In

H.K. and S.K. contributed equally to this work.

KARGER

Fax +41 61 306 12 34
E-Mail karger@karger.ch
www.karger.com

1018–2438/10/1525–0047$26.00/0

Accessible online at:
www.karger.com/iaa

Correspondence to: Dr. Shin-ichiro Kagami or Dr. Hiroshi Nakajima
Department of Molecular Genetics, Graduate School of Medicine
Chiba University, 1-8-1 Inohana
Chiba City, Chiba 260-8670 (Japan)
Tel. +81 43 226 2197, Fax +81 43 226 2199, E-Mail kagams@faculty.chiba-u.jp

Table 1. Characteristics of the patients with LGE and increased IgG4 levels

Patient	Age/sex	Enlargement	IgG4 mg/dl (%)	IgE IU/ml	Ag-IgE (class)	EOS n/μl	IgG4+ cells	Wheezing	Complications
1	36/M	L(b), S	223 (18.8)	450	negative	638	ND	+	
2	44/M	L(b)	300 (17.4)	205	negative	112	+		
3	56/M	L(b)	159 (9.4)	447	JC(4)	130	ND		
4	67/M	L(b), S	963 (29.2)	407	negative	863	+		
5	68/M	L	1,600 (34.4)	585	negative	496	+		
6	73/M	L(b)	723 (25.7)	358	negative	622	+	+	RPF
7	63/F	L(b), S	916 (27.9)	570	negative	402	+	+	AIP
8	64/F	L(b)	3,280 (33.0)	1,133	negative	159	+	+	AIP
9	65/F	L(b), P(b)	855 (29.9)	984	negative	51	ND	+	

IgG4 (%) = Serum IgG4/total serum IgG ratio; Ag-IgE = allergen-specific IgE; EOS = blood eosinophil counts; IgG4+ cells = prominent infiltration of IgG4-bearing plasmacytes in lacrimal glands; L = lacrimal gland; P = parotid gland; S = submandibular gland; (b) = bilateral; JC = Japanese cedar pollen; ND = not determined; RPF = retroperitoneal fibrosis; AIP = autoimmune pancreatitis.

addition, MD patients show marked serum IgG4 elevation and infiltration of plasmacytes expressing IgG4 in the enlarged exocrine glands, whereas SjS patients show no elevation in serum IgG4.

In addition to MD, it has been reported that the serum IgG4 elevation is associated with several clinical conditions [5], e.g. autoimmune pancreatitis [6], sclerosing cholangitis [7], retroperitoneal fibrosis [8], tubulointerstitial nephritis [9] and inflammatory pseudotumour of the lung [10]. Moreover, IgG4-related diseases such as retroperitoneal fibrosis and tubulointerstitial nephritis are occasionally accompanied by MD [3]. Based on these findings, Masaki et al. [11] proposed a new clinical entity for IgG4-related plasmacytic syndrome comprising autoimmune pancreatitis, retroperitoneal fibrosis and MD. Regarding the pathogenesis of IgG4-related plasmacytic syndrome, Th2 cells have been reported to be increased at the site of IgG4-related autoimmune pancreatitis [12]. More recently, a case of IgG4-related MD with enhanced Th2 cytokine production was reported [13]. However, the role of Th2 cells and their cytokines in the pathogenesis of IgG4-related diseases is still largely unknown.

To unravel the pathogenesis of IgG4-related diseases, we evaluated the clinical characteristics, and cytokine expression and differentiation of CD4+ T cells in patients with IgG4-related lacrimal gland enlargement (LGE). In the majority of our patients, serum IgE was elevated and about half of the patients presented eosinophilia and asthma-like symptoms. Th2 cytokines and GATA-3, a master regulator of Th2 cells [14], on CD4+ T cells were increased in patients compared with healthy controls. CD4+ T cells from the patients also expressed increased levels of IL-10, which has been shown to enhance IgG4 production [15, 16], compared with healthy controls. These findings suggest the possible involvement of Th2 cells and IL-10 in the pathogenesis of IgG4-related diseases.

Patients and Methods

Patients

Nine patients with LGE and increased serum IgG4 levels (>135 mg/dl, named IgG4-related LGE) were enrolled in this study between June 2007 and May 2009 in Chiba University Hospital, Chiba, Japan. None of the patients with IgG4-related LGE were treated with oral corticosteroids at examination. The clinical characteristics of the patients are shown in table 1. Age-matched atopic asthma patients were randomly enrolled from the database of the Chiba University Hospital (n = 10). Asthmatic patients were taking inhaled budesonide or fluticasone, but none of them took oral corticosteroids. Age-matched patients with primary SjS who were diagnosed according to the revised criteria of the American-European Consensus Group [17] were retrieved from the database of Chiba University Hospital (n = 10) and also included in the study. None of the SjS patients took oral corticosteroids. Healthy controls with no history of atopic or autoimmune diseases (serum IgE <100 U/ml) and negative results for anti-nuclear antibody were also examined (n = 5). The study design was approved by the Ethics Committee of Chiba University (No. 396), and informed consent was obtained from each patient before study enrollment.

Isolation of CD4+ T Cells and Cell Culture

CD4+ T cells were isolated from the peripheral blood of patients with IgG4-related LGE (patients 1, 4, 6, 8 and 9), atopic asthma patients (n = 5) and healthy controls (n = 5). Briefly, mononuclear cells were isolated from the peripheral blood by Ficoll-Paque density gradient centrifugation. Mononuclear cells were stained with biotin-conjugated anti-CD4 monoclonal antibody (mAb) and then with anti-biotin microbeads according to the manufacturer's instruction (CD4+ T-cell isolation kit II; Miltenyi Biotec, Sunnyvale, Calif., USA). The resultant cells were >98% pure CD4+ T cells by FACS analysis. Purified CD4+ T cells were stimulated with plate-bound anti-CD3 mAb (OKT3, 1 μg/ml; eBioscience, San Diego, Calif., USA) plus anti-CD28 mAb (2 μg/ml, eBioscience) in RPMI-1640 medium supplemented with 10% heat-inactivated fetal calf serum, 2 mM L-glutamine, and antibiotics at 37°C. Six days later, cells were re-stimulated with plate-bound anti-CD3 mAb for 24 h and then harvested.

Real-Time PCR Analysis

Total cellular RNA was extracted with ISOGEN solution (Nippon Gene, Tokyo, Japan). Reverse transcription was carried out using an iScript cDNA synthesis kit (Bio-Rad, Hercules, Calif., USA). Expression of IL-4, IL-5, IL-10, IL-13, IL-21, IFN-γ, GATA-3 and T-bet was determined by real-time quantitative PCR using a standard protocol on ABI PRISM 7300 instrument (Applied Biosystems, Foster City, Calif., USA). The levels of IL-4, IL-5, IL-10, IL-13, IL-21, IFN-γ, GATA-3 and T-bet were normalized to the levels of β-actin.

Data Analysis

Data are summarized as means ± SD. Statistical analyses of the results were performed by the unpaired t test or by the Pearson correlation test; $p < 0.05$ was considered significantly different.

Results

Characteristics of the Patients with LGE and Increased IgG4 Levels

Nine patients with LGE and increased serum IgG4 levels (IgG4-related LGE) were enrolled in this study between June 2007 and May 2009 at the Chiba University Hospital. Six of the 9 patients were male, and mean age was 59.6 years (range 36–73 years; table 1). Eight patients had bilateral LGE and 3 patients also had submandibular gland swelling (table 1). IgG4 levels, which were determined by standard nephelometry (SRL, Tokyo, Japan), were much higher in patients with IgG4-related LGE than in patients with SjS and atopic asthma or healthy controls (n = 9–10, $p < 0.01$; fig. 1a). The levels of IgG1 in patients with IgG4-related LGE were similar to those in SjS patients but were higher than those in patients with atopic asthma or healthy controls ($p < 0.05$; fig. 1a). The levels of IgG2 tended to be higher in patients with IgG4-related LGE than in patients with SjS or atopic asthma (fig. 1a). All patients with IgG4-related LGE as well as those with atopic asthma were negative for anti-SS-A antibody, whereas 9 of 10 SjS patients were positive for anti-SS-A antibody. Histological analyses of lacrimal glands were performed on 6 patients with IgG4-related LGE, and all of the biopsy specimens showed prominent infiltration of IgG4-bearing plasmacytes (IgG4+/IgG+ plasma cell ratio >0.5; table 1). The following complications were reported: autoimmune pancreatitis in 2 patients with IgG4-related LGE and retroperitoneal fibrosis in 1 patient (table 1).

Serum IgE Levels and Blood Eosinophil Counts Are Elevated in Patients with IgG4-Related LGE

Similar to IgE, IgG4 production is induced by IL-4 and IL-13 [18]. In addition, IgG4 is produced in part as an intermediate product during sequential switching from IgM to IgE [18, 19]. We then examined serum IgE levels in patients with IgG4-related LGE. Interestingly, all patients with IgG4-related LGE exhibited elevated IgE levels (>170 IU/ml) and the levels were comparable to those in patients with atopic asthma (fig. 1b; table 1). The number of peripheral blood eosinophils was also increased (>400/μl) in 5 of 9 patients with IgG4-related LGE (table 1). Comparison of IgG4 levels with IgE levels in the patients yielded a correlation coefficient of 0.75 (n = 9, $p < 0.05$; fig. 1c), but blood eosinophil counts were not correlated with the level of IgG4 (fig. 1d). CAP FEIA (fluorescence immunoassay) revealed that although 1 patient had allergen-specific IgE against Japanese cedar pollen, a most common allergen for seasonal allergic rhinitis in Japan, the other 8 patients did not have allergen-specific IgE against 10 inhaled allergens tested, including house dust mites *(Dermatophagoides farinae)*, cat dander, grass pollen, Japanese cedar pollen and four molds (SRL, Tokyo, Japan; table 1).

Interestingly, consistent with increased serum IgE levels and blood eosinophilia, 5 of 9 patients with IgG4-related LGE developed asthma-like symptoms, such as wheezing and persistent cough (table 1) with normal chest radiography, although they had not been diagnosed as having asthma. Inhalation of β_2-agonist increased FEV_1 and was effective against wheezing in patients with IgG4-related LGE, confirming the reversibility of airway narrowing.

Increased Production of Th2 Cytokines and GATA-3 Expression on CD4+ T Cells in Patients with IgG4-Related LGE

Because serum IgE levels as well as blood eosinophil counts were increased in patients with IgG4-related LGE, we next examined mRNA expression of Th2 cytokines as well as GATA-3 on CD4+ T cells in the patients. As shown

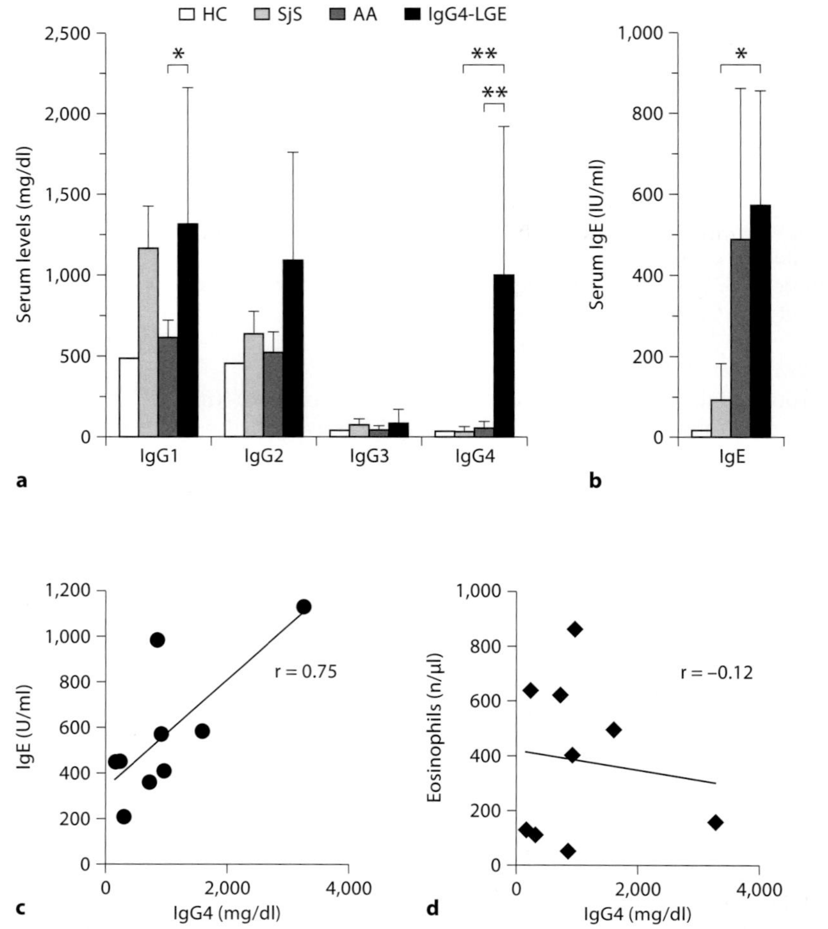

Fig. 1. Serum IgE levels are increased in patients with IgG4-related LGE. Serum levels of IgG1, IgG2, IgG3, IgG4 (**a**) and IgE (**b**) in patients with IgG4-related LGE (IgG4-LGE; n = 9), SjS (n = 10) and atopic asthma (AA; n = 10), and in Japanese healthy controls (HC; only mean data; provided by SRL) were examined by standard nephelometry. Means ± SD, * $p < 0.05$, ** $p < 0.01$. **c, d** Serum IgG4 levels correlate with serum IgE levels but not with blood eosinophil counts in patients with IgG4-related LGE. Serum IgG4 levels and either serum IgE levels (**c**) or blood eosinophil counts (**d**) were plotted in patients with IgG4-related LGE. Comparison of serum IgG4 versus serum IgE levels yielded a correlation coefficient of 0.75 (n = 9, $p < 0.05$).

in figure 2a, b, IL-4 and IL-5 expression was significantly increased in patients with IgG4-related LGE compared with healthy controls (n = 5, each, $p < 0.05$). Although there was no statistical difference, the levels of IL-4, IL-5 and IL-13 tended to be increased in patients with IgG4-related LGE compared with atopic asthma patients (fig. 2a–c). IL-10, which has been shown to enhance IL-4-induced IgG4 production [15], was also significantly increased on CD4+ T cells in patients with IgG4-related LGE compared with healthy controls (n = 5, $p < 0.05$; fig. 2d). In contrast, IL-21, which also enhances IL-4-induced IgG4 production [20, 21], was not significantly increased in patients with IgG4-related LGE (fig. 2e). The expression of GATA-3, a master regulator of Th2 cells [14], but not T-bet, a master regulator of Th1 cells [22], was also higher on CD4+ T cells in patients with IgG4-related LGE than in healthy controls (n = 5, $p < 0.05$; fig. 2g, h). These results suggest that clinical characteristics of patients with IgG4-related LGE, such as elevated IgG4 and IgE levels and eosinophilia, may be accounted for by the enhanced Th2 cell differentiation and IL-10 production.

Discussion

In this study, we examined the clinical characteristics and the profile of peripheral blood CD4+ T cells in patients with IgG4-related LGE. All patients with IgG4-related LGE had elevated serum IgE levels (table 1; fig. 1b) and about half of the patients with IgG4-related LGE exhibited eosinophilia and asthma-like symptoms (table 1). In addition, Th2 cell differentiation and IL-10 production of peripheral blood CD4+ T cells were enhanced in the

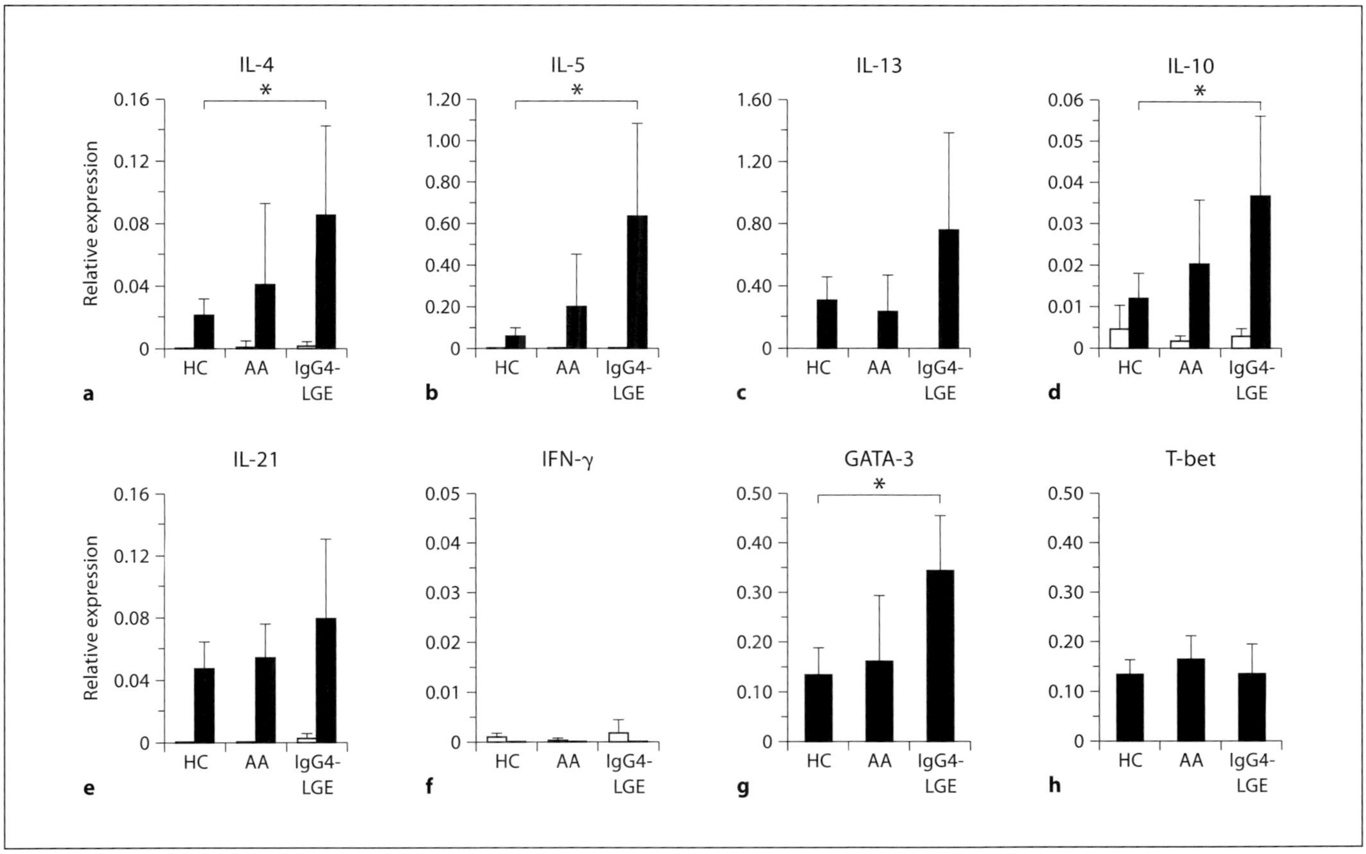

Fig. 2. The expression of Th2 cytokines and GATA-3 is elevated in patients with IgG4-related LGE. CD4+ T cells from patients with IgG4-related LGE (n = 5) and atopic asthma (AA; n = 5), and healthy controls (HC; n = 5) were stimulated with plate-bound anti-CD3 mAb plus anti-CD28 mAb. Six days later, cells were re-stimulated with plate-bound anti-CD3 mAb for 24 h, and the levels of IL-4 (**a**), IL-5 (**b**), IL-10 (**d**), IL-13 (**c**), IL-21 (**e**) and IFN-γ (**f**) as well as GATA-3 (**g**) and T-bet (**h**) were analyzed by real-time PCR and normalized to those of β-actin. Means ± SD, n = 5 each, * $p < 0.05$.

patients (fig. 2). These findings suggest the possible involvement of Th2 cells in the pathogenesis of IgG4-related LGE.

In addition, the levels of IgE are significantly correlated with those of IgG4 (fig. 1c). Consistent with the enhanced IgE production and eosinophilia in the patients, the production of Th2 cytokines, e.g. IL-4 and IL-5, and GATA-3 expression on CD4+ T cells is increased in the patients (fig. 2). Recently, Miyake et al. [13] have also reported a case of MD with elevated IgE levels, eosinophilia and an elevated Th2 cytokine expression in peripheral blood mononuclear cells. These findings suggest that Th2 cells are involved in the pathogenesis of IgG4-related diseases. Importantly, consistent with these findings, about half of the patients with IgG4-related LGE complained of asthma-like symptoms (table 1), with reversibility of airway narrowing in response to β_2-agonist inhalation. These findings suggest that stimulation with unidentified airborne allergens rather than bystander activation of B cells may induce Th2 cell activation and IgE production and subsequent asthma-like symptoms in patients with IgG4-related LGE.

It is well known that both IgE and IgG4 are induced by IL-4 and IL-13 upon stimulation with allergens [19, 23]. Although serum IgE levels are elevated in both atopic asthma patients and patients with IgG4-related LGE, the IgG4/IgE ratio is much higher in patients with IgG4-related LGE (fig. 1a, b), suggesting that in addition to IL-4 and/or IL-13, some other factors may also be involved in the increased IgG4 production in patients with IgG4-related LGE. In this regard, a previous work has shown that the high IFN-γ/IL-4 ratio is associated with IgG4 production in MD [3]. In addition, we show here that the expression of IL-10, which enhances IL-4-induced IgG4 production [15, 16], is elevated on CD4+ T cells in patients with IgG4-related LGE (fig. 2d). In contrast, the expression of IL-21, which also enhances IL-4-induced IgG4 production [20, 21], is not significantly elevated in the patients (fig. 2e). Enhanced IL-10 expression was also reported at the site of IgG4-related sclerosing pancreatitis [12]. Taken together, it is suggested that in addition to IL-4 and/or IL-13, enhanced production of IL-10 may be involved in the elevated IgG4/IgE ratio in patients with IgG4-related LGE and that IL-10 could be a novel therapeutic target for patients with IgG4-related diseases.

Regarding the clonality of IgG4-producing cells in IgG4-related diseases, Yamada et al. [24] have recently demonstrated that most IgG4-positive cells infiltrating lacrimal glands and the peripheral blood are polyclonal. In addition, somatic hypermutation of IgG4-positive plasma cells was noted in lacrimal glands in MD [24]. These findings suggest an antigen-driven local immune response in IgG4-related diseases. Because IgE-producing plasma cells can develop in part from IgG4-producing B cells by sequential switching [18, 19], antigen specificity of IgE antibodies in the patients seems to be overlapping with the specificity of IgG4 antibodies. Identification of allergen that causes asthma-like symptoms in IgG4-related LGE may provide some clues to the pathogenesis of IgG4-related diseases.

In conclusion, we show that Th2 cytokines and IL-10 production on CD4+ T cells are enhanced in patients with IgG4-related LGE, and that about half of our patients with IgG4-related LGE develop asthma-like symptoms. Although further studies are necessary to elucidate the molecular basis of our findings, our results add new insights into the pathogenesis of IgG4-related diseases.

Acknowledgments

This work was supported in part by grants-in-aids for scientific research from the Ministry of Education, Culture, Sports, Science and Technology, the Japanese Government and by the Global COE Program (Global Center for Education and Research in Immune System Regulation and Treatment), MEXT, Japan.

Disclosure Statement

The authors declare that no financial or other conflict of interest exists in relation to the content of this article.

References

1 Morgan WS, Castleman B: A clinicopathologic study of Mikulicz's disease. Am J Pathol 1953;29:471–503.

2 Yamamoto M, Ohara M, Suzuki C, Naishiro Y, Yamamoto H, Takahashi H, Imai K: Elevated IgG4 concentrations in serum of patients with Mikulicz's disease. Scand J Rheumatol 2004;33:432–433.

3 Yamamoto M, Harada S, Ohara M, Suzuki C, Naishiro Y, Yamamoto H, Takahashi H, Imai K: Clinical and pathological differences between Mikulicz's disease and Sjögren's syndrome. Rheumatology 2005;44:227–234.

4 Yoshimoto M, Takahashi H, Ohara M, Suzuki C, Naishiro Y, Yamamoto H, Shinomura Y, Imai K: A new conceptualization for Mikulicz's disease as an IgG4-related plasmacytic disease. Mod Rheumatol 2006;16: 335–340.

5 Neild GH, Rodriguez-Justo M, Wall C, Connolly JO: Hyper-IgG4 disease: report and characterisation of a new disease. BMC Med 2006;4:23.

6 Hamano H, Kawa S, Horiuchi A, Unno H, Furuya N, Akamatsu T, Fukushima M, Nikaido T, Nakayama K, Usuda N, Kiyosawa K: High serum IgG4 concentrations in patients with sclerosing pancreatitis. N Engl J Med 2001;344:732–738.

7 Ichimura T, Kondo S, Ambo Y, Hirano S, Ohmi M, Okushiba S, Morikawa T, Shimizu M, Katoh H: Primary sclerosing cholangitis associated with autoimmune pancreatitis. Hepatogastroenterology 2002; 49: 1221–1224.

8 Hamano H, Kawa S, Ochi Y, Unno H, Shiba N, Wajiki M, Nakazawa K, Shimojo H, Kiyosawa K: Hydronephrosis associated with retroperitoneal fibrosis and sclerosing pancreatitis. Lancet 2002;359:1403–1404.

9 Takeda S, Haratake J, Kasai T, Takaeda C, Takazakura E: IgG4-associated idiopathic tubulointerstitial nephritis complicating autoimmune pancreatitis. Nephrol Dial Transplant 2004;19:474–476.

10 Zen Y, Kitagawa S, Minato H, Kurumaya H, Katayanagi K, Masuda S, Niwa H, Fujimura M, Nakanuma Y: IgG4-positive plasma cells in inflammatory pseudotumor (plasma cell granuloma) of the lung. Hum Pathol 2005; 36:710–717.

11 Masaki Y, Dong L, Kurose N, Kitagawa K, Morikawa Y, Yamamoto M, Takahashi H, Shinomura Y, Imai K, Saeki T, Azumi A, Nakada S, Sugiyama E, Matsui S, Origuchi T, Nishiyama S, Nishimori I, Nojima T, Yamada K, Kawano M, Zen Y, Kaneko M, Miyazaki K, Tsubota K, Eguchi K, Tomoda K, Sawaki T, Kawanami T, Tanaka M, Fukushima T, Sugai S, Umehara H: Proposal for a new clinical entity, IgG4-positive multiorgan lymphoproliferative syndrome: analysis of 64 cases of IgG4-related disorders. Ann Rheum Dis 2009;68:1310–1315.

12 Zen Y, Fujii T, Harada K, Kawano M, Yamada K, Takahira M, Nakanuma Y: Th2 and regulatory immune reactions are increased in immunoglobulin IgG4-related sclerosing pancreatitis and cholangitis. Hepatology 2007;45:1538–1546.

13 Miyake K, Moriyama M, Aizawa K, Nagano S, Inoue Y, Sadanaga A, Nakashima H, Nakamura S: Peripheral CD4+ T cells showing a Th2 phenotype in a patient with Mikulicz's disease associated with lymphadenopathy and pleural effusion. Mod Rheumatol 2008; 18:86–90.

14 Zheng W, Flavell RA: The transcription factor GATA-3 is necessary and sufficient for Th2 cytokine gene expression in CD4 T cells. Cell 1997;89:587–596.

15 Jeannin P, Lecoanet S, Delneste Y, Gauchat JF, Bonnefoy JY: IgE versus IgG4 production can be differentially regulated by IL-10. J Immunol 1998;160:3555–3561.

16 Satoguina JS, Weyand E, Larbi J, Hoerauf A: T regulatory-1 cells induce IgG4 production by B cells: role of IL-10. J Immunol 2005;174: 4718–4726.
17 Vitali C, Bombardieri S, Jonsson R, Moutsopoulos HM, Alexander EL, Carsons SE, Daniels TE, Fox PC, Fox RI, Kassan SS, Pillemer SR, Talal N, Weisman MH, European Study Group on Classification Criteria for Sjögren's Syndrome: Classification criteria for Sjögren's syndrome: a revised version of the European criteria proposed by the American-European Consensus Group. Ann Rheum Dis 2002;61:554–558.
18 Aalberse RC, Stapel SO, Schuurman J, Rispens T: Immunoglobulin G4: an odd antibody. Clin Exp Allergy 2009;39:469–477.
19 Jabara HH, Loh R, Ramesh N, Vercelli D, Geha RS: Sequential switching from μ to ε via $\gamma 4$ in human B cells stimulated with IL-4 and hydrocortisone. J Immunol 1993;151: 4528–4533.
20 Wood N, Bourque K, Donaldson DD, Collins M, Vercelli D, Goldman SJ, Kasaian MT: IL-21 effects on human IgE production in response to IL-4 or IL-13. Cell Immunol 2004; 231:133–145.
21 Avery DT, Bryant VL, Ma CS, de Waal MR, Tangye SG: IL-21-induced isotype switching to IgG and IgA by human naive B cells is differentially regulated by IL-4. J Immunol 2008;181:1767–1779.
22 Szabo SJ, Kim ST, Costa GL, Zhang X, Fathman CG, Glimcher LH: A novel transcription factor, T-bet, directs Th1 lineage commitment. Cell 2000;100:655–669.
23 Punnonen J, Aversa G, Cocks BG, McKenzie AN, Menon S, Zurawski G, de Waal Malefyt R, de Vries JE: Interleukin 13 induces interleukin 4-independent IgG4 and IgE synthesis and CD23 expression by human B cells. Proc Natl Acad Sci USA 1993;15:3730–3734.
24 Yamada K, Kawano M, Inoue R, Hamano R, Kakuchi Y, Fujii H, Matsumura M, Zen Y, Takahira M, Yachie A, Yamagishi M: Clonal relationship between infiltrating immunoglobulin G4 (IgG4)-positive plasma cells in lacrimal glands and circulating IgG4-positive lymphocytes in Mikulicz's disease. Clin Exp Immunol 2008;152:432–439.

Original Paper

International Archives of Allergy and Immunology

Int Arch Allergy Immunol 2010;152(suppl 1):54–61
DOI: 10.1159/000312126

Published online: June 4, 2010

Basophil Activation Marker CD203c Is Useful in the Diagnosis of Hen's Egg and Cow's Milk Allergies in Children

Sakura Sato[a] Hiroshi Tachimoto[b] Akinori Shukuya[b] Norimasa Kurosaka[b] Noriyuki Yanagida[b] Tomohiro Utsunomiya[b] Masamichi Iguchi[b] Takatsugu Komata[b] Takanori Imai[b] Morimitsu Tomikawa[b] Motohiro Ebisawa[a]

[a]Clinical Research Center for Allergy and Rheumatology and [b]Department of Pediatrics, Sagamihara National Hospital, Sagamihara, Japan

Key Words

Basophil activation test · CD203c · Egg allergy · Food allergy · Milk allergy · Oral food challenge test

Abstract

Background: The diagnosis of food allergy (FA) is usually based on oral food challenge tests (OFC). However, OFCs occasionally induce severe adverse reactions. CD203c expression on basophils is emerging as a potential diagnostic index. We evaluated whether CD203c expression on basophils would be a useful marker of OFC-associated symptoms in hen's egg and cow's milk allergies in children. ***Methods:*** Seventy-one patients who had been diagnosed with FA based on OFCs or a convincing history of FA symptoms in the Department of Pediatrics, Sagamihara National Hospital, were recruited. CD203c expression was assessed after stimulation with antigens (egg white, ovomucoid, milk or casein) using allergenicity kits. The CD203c stimulation index (SI = the allergen-induced CD203c expression level divided by the baseline expression level) and the threshold of CD203c expression (the minimum concentration of antigen to induce CD203c SI ≥2) were analyzed in association with tolerance acquisition. ***Results:*** For the CD203c SI, the areas under the receiver-operating characteristic curve were 0.72 for egg white, 0.82 for ovomucoid, 0.84 for milk and 0.67 for casein. The positive predictive value for the threshold of CD203c expression was 94.7% for egg white, 100% for ovomucoid, 85.7% for milk and 75.0% for casein. ***Conclusions:*** Assessment of food antigen-induced CD203c expression on basophils is useful to determine if children will outgrow FA as well as in decision making regarding whether or not to perform OFCs.

Introduction

The definitive diagnosis of food allergy (FA) is generally based on oral food challenge tests (OFC). Since OFCs occasionally induce severe reactions, whether or not to perform OFCs should be carefully considered. Antigen-specific IgE levels, a useful predictor of OFC-associated symptoms, have been widely used in clinical practice [1–4]. However, antigen-specific IgE is highly sensitive but less specific, and the development of more reliable tests for FA diagnosis has been sought.

When a causative antigen is bound to specific IgE on the surface of the cell membrane of a basophil, cross-linking of the high-affinity IgE receptor (FcεRI) occurs, inducing the release of histamine and the production of leukotrienes and cytokines. Because of this mechanism,

KARGER

Fax +41 61 306 12 34
E-Mail karger@karger.ch
www.karger.com

1018–2438/10/1525–0054$26.00/0

Accessible online at:
www.karger.com/iaa

Correspondence to: Dr. Motohiro Ebisawa
Clinical Research Center for Allergy and Rheumatology
Sagamihara National Hospital
18-1, Sakuradai, Sagamihara-City, Kanagawa 228-8522 (Japan)
Tel. +81 42 742 8311, Fax +81 42 742 5314, E-Mail m-ebisawa@sagamihara-hosp.gr.jp

peripheral blood basophils have been employed in tests, such as the histamine release test, to identify specific antigens that induce type I hypersensitivity [5].

A basophil activation test (BAT) determines CD63 and CD203c expression on basophils using flow cytometry. Recently, BATs have been reported to be useful in the diagnosis of IgE-dependent allergies [6, 7] and have been evaluated in association with a variety of different allergies [8–12].

CD203c (also called ectonucleotide pyrophosphatase/phosphodiesterase 3; E-NPP3) is an ecto-enzyme consisting of 875 amino acids belonging to a family of ectonucleotide pyrophosphatases and phosphodiesterases [13, 14]. It is expressed on the cell membrane of human peripheral basophils and mast cells [14, 15], and cross-linking of the high-affinity IgE receptor up-regulates CD203c expression on the cell membrane [11, 12]. In a previous study, CD203c expression was up-regulated following antigen stimulation in patients with bee venom [12] and grass pollen allergies [11], as well as after immunotherapy in patients with a history of systemic reactions to bee venom [9]. The sensitivity and specificity of antigen-induced CD203c expression were reported to be 75 and 100%, respectively, in the diagnosis of latex allergy [8]. More recently, Tokuda et al. [16] and Ocmant et al. [17] published papers on the utility of food antigen-induced CD203c expression in the diagnosis of FA. Ocmant et al. [17] reported that sensitivity and specificity of ovalbumin (OVA)-induced BATs applied to diagnose egg allergy were 62.5 and 96.4, respectively. Consequently, BATs may be beneficial in the diagnosis of FA. In the study by Tokuda et al. [16], measurement of purified native ω-5 gliadin-induced enhancement of CD203c on basophils is useful for the diagnosis of immediate wheat allergy in children. In the present study, we evaluated whether CD203c expression on basophils induced by food antigen would be useful in the prediction of OFC-associated symptoms in hen's egg and milk allergies.

Patients and Methods

Patients

Seventy-one patients (49 males and 22 females aged 6.6 ± 3.2 years, mean ± SD) who had previously been diagnosed with FA and had been followed up in our hospital (Division of Pediatrics, Sagamihara National Hospital) between July 2006 and October 2007 were recruited to this study. Acquisition of food tolerance was diagnosed based on the results of OFCs or a convincing history of symptoms after food ingestion during the 6 months before or after sample collection.

Grouping of Subjects Based on the Acquisition of Food Tolerance

Of all subjects, those who were tested for simultaneous measurement of CD203c expression and antigen-specific IgE were grouped as follows: for egg allergy, subjects with heated- and raw-egg allergy who reacted after ingestion of heated and raw eggs (HEA+/REA+), those without heated-egg allergy and raw-egg allergy who did not develop symptoms after ingestion of heated eggs but reacted after ingestion of raw eggs (HEA–/REA+), and those without heated- and raw-egg allergy who did not develop symptoms after ingestion of heated and raw eggs (HEA–/REA–); for milk allergy, subjects with milk allergy (MA+) who developed symptoms after drinking milk and those without milk allergy (MA–) who did not develop symptoms after drinking milk. The number of subjects tested depended on the antigens used as follows: for stimulation by egg white, 38 subjects with HEA+/REA+ versus 5 with (HEA–/REA+) versus 8 with (HEA–/REA–); for stimulation by ovomucoid, 35 versus 5 versus 6; for stimulation with milk, 27 with MA+ versus 23 with MA–, and for stimulation by casein, 21 versus 17. Areas under the curve (AUCs) were determined by receiver-operating characteristic (ROC) analysis to evaluate the utility of CD203c on basophils in determining the outgrowing of FA. The sensitivity, specificity, positive predictive value (PPV), negative predictive value (NPV) and efficiency of the CD203 stimulation index (SI) and the threshold of CD203c were also determined.

Measurement of CD203c Expression on Peripheral Blood Basophils

CD203c expression on peripheral blood basophils was assessed using the Allergenicity Kit (Beckman Coulter, Fullerton, Calif., USA) on the day of sample collection. First, whole blood was drawn into plastic tubes containing EDTA 2Na (100 μl), 20 μl of antigen, and 20 μl of tricolored antibodies (CRTH2-FITC, CD203c-PE and CD3-PC7) and 100 μl of activation buffer were mixed in a plastic tube. The mixture was then incubated at 37°C for 15 min. After incubation, 100 μl of stop solution was added to stop the reaction, as well as lysis-fixing solution, and the mixture was incubated for 10 min at room temperature. The mixture was centrifuged at 200 *g* for 5 min, and the supernatant was aspirated. The sample was washed with phosphate-buffered saline, fixed with 0.1% formaldehyde, and then assayed by flow cytometry. The following antigens were used: anti-IgE antibody (Beckman Coulter), egg white, milk (Greer Laboratories, Lenoir, N.C., USA), ovomucoid (trypsin inhibitor from purified hen egg white ovomucoid type III-0, No. T-2011, Sigma-Aldrich, St. Louis, Mo., USA) and casein (α-casein; Sigma-Aldrich). The antigen concentrations used were as follows: 1,000 ng/ml for anti-IgE antibody, and 0.1, 10 and 1,000 ng/ml were employed for egg white, milk, ovomucoid and casein. CD203c expression on basophils was assessed using geometric mean fluorescence intensity. Antigen-induced CD203c expression was calculated using the formula of 'the antigen-induced CD203c expression – the baseline CD203c expression,' and the maximum CD203c expression was defined as the highest expression. The CD203c SI was defined as the antigen-induced CD203c expression divided by the baseline CD203c expression [11], and the threshold of CD203c expression was defined as the minimum concentration of an antigen that produces CD203c SI ≥2.

Oral Food Challenges

Oral food challenges were performed in an open challenge or single-blinded challenge [18]. In the open-challenge test, the hen's egg challenge test was performed using heated whole egg (about 30 g), and 35 g of yogurt or 200 ml of milk was used for the milk challenge test. In single-blinded challenges, freeze-dried powder of raw egg or milk (QP Institute, Tokyo, Japan) was used [19]. In an OFC, the patient initially ingested 1/16 of the total challenge dose of allergenic food and, subsequently, ingested increasing portions at an interval of 15 min until finishing the total challenge dose in 1 h. The patient was monitored until 24 h after food ingestion. If symptoms developed during the OFC, the test was terminated and the patient was carefully monitored. If the patient tested negative or slightly positive, ingestion of causative food at home was checked at every hospital visit to determine the patient was outgrowing the FA.

Antigen-Specific IgE Antibodies

Antigen-specific IgE antibodies against egg white, ovomucoid, milk and casein were determined by the CAP System FEIA (Phadia, Uppsala, Sweden) on the day of CD203c measurement or within 6 months before or after. The detection limit of the assay was 0.35 kUa/l.

Statistical Analysis

Results were presented as means ± SD or means ± SEM. Comparisons of groups were performed using the Mann-Whitney U test and the χ^2 test. For multiple comparisons, one-way analysis of variance followed by Dunn's multiple-comparison test was employed. $p < 0.05$ was considered statistically significant. ROC curve analyses were performed to analyze CD203c SI induced by food antigens, and the highest levels of sensitivity and specificity were used as cutoff values. They were calculated using GraphPad Prism (version 5).

Results

Characteristics of the patients are summarized in table 1. The average age did not significantly differ between patients with egg allergy and those with milk allergy. The average antigen-specific IgE level was significantly higher in the HEA+/REA+ group than in other egg allergy groups and in the MA+ group than in the other milk group.

The baseline CD203c expression level was 331.1 ± 46.0 (mean ± SEM) for the HEA+/REA+ group, 385.6 ± 137.8 for the HEA–/REA+ group and 245.7 ± 41.9 for the HEA–/REA– group (nonsignificant). The baseline CD203c expression was 302.1 ± 33.9 for the MA+ group and 332.5 ± 62.2 for the MA– group (nonsignificant). No significant difference was observed between groups with egg and milk allergies.

As shown in figure 1a, the maximum CD203c expression induced by egg white was 755.5 ± 86.1 (mean ± SEM) for the HEA+/REA+ group, 422.6 ± 218.2 for the HEA–/REA+ group and 293.7 ± 100.2 for the HEA–/REA– group (nonsignificant). The CD203c SI was 4.2 ± 0.4 for the HEA+/REA+ group, 2.3 ± 0.4 for the HEA–/REA+ group and 2.3 ± 0.5 for the HEA–/REA– group (nonsignificant). Although average CD203c expression was increased in the HEA+/REA+ group, the difference was not significant between egg allergy groups. On the other hand, the maximum CD203c expression level induced by ovomucoid was 727.7 ± 102.0 for the HEA+/REA+ group, 325.9 ± 204.1 for the HEA–/REA+ group and 108.5 ± 32.1 for the HEA–/REA– group, i.e. CD203c expression was significantly increased in the HEA+/REA+ group ($p < 0.05$). The CD203c SI was 3.8 ± 0.4 for the HEA+/REA+ group, 2.0 ± 0.4 for the HEA–/REA+ group and 1.4 ± 0.1 for the HEA–/REA– group, demonstrating that CD203c SI was significantly higher in the HEA+/REA+ group ($p < 0.05$).

As shown in figure 1b, the maximum CD203c expression induced by milk was 944.4 ± 136.2 for the MA+ group and 273.4 ± 105.1 for the MA– group, and the CD203c SI was 4.5 ± 0.5 for the MA+ group and 1.9 ± 0.4 for the MA– group, i.e. both parameters were significantly higher in the MA+ group ($p < 0.05$). The maxi-

Table 1. Patient profiles

	HEA+/REA+	HEA–/REA+	HEA–/REA–
Egg white (n = 51)			
Patients, n	38	5	8
Average age, years	6.5 ± 3.1	5.5 ± 2.3	7.7 ± 4.4
Antigen-specific IgE, Ua/ml	21.8 ± 24.8*	5.0 ± 6.5	3.3 ± 3.7
Ovomucoid (n = 46)			
Patients, n	35	5	6
Average age, years	6.6 ± 3.2	5.5 ± 2.3	8.3 ± 4.9
Antigen-specific IgE, Ua/ml	16.3 ± 25.0*	2.5 ± 2.4	3.4 ± 3.5
	MA+	MA–	
Milk (n = 50)			
Patients, n	27	23	
Average age, years	6.5 ± 3.4	6.3 ± 2.9	
Antigen-specific IgE, Ua/ml	22.5 ± 32.5*	6.3 ± 11.1	
Casein (n = 38)			
Patients, n	21	17	
Average age, years	7.6 ± 3.5	6.4 ± 3.0	
Antigen-specific IgE, Ua/ml	17.8 ± 24.9*	7.6 ± 13.3	

* p <0.05, Mann-Whitney U test.

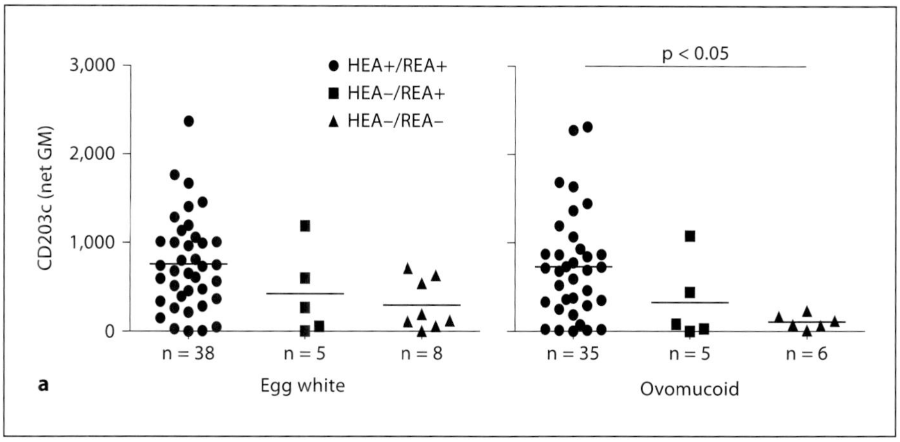

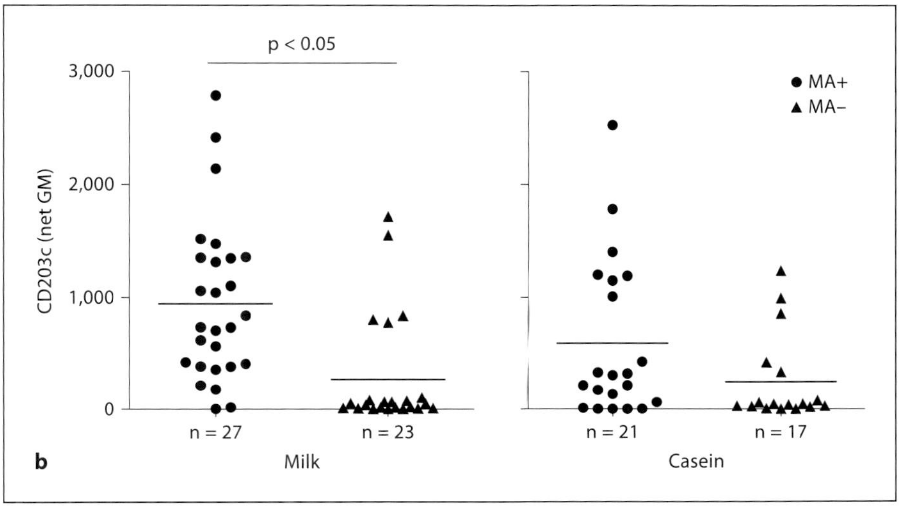

Fig. 1. Relationships between FA diagnosis and CD203c expression on basophils in patients with hen's egg allergy (**a**) and cow's milk allergy (**b**). * $p < 0.05$, Dunn's multiple comparison test. GM = Geometric mean fluorescence intensity.

mum CD203c expression level induced by casein was 592.4 ± 153.5 for the MA+ group and 248.2 ± 95.6 for the MA– group, and the CD203c SI was 3.1 ± 0.5 for the MA+ group and 1.7 ± 0.3 for the MA– group, with no significant difference between the groups.

ROC analyses were performed for CD203c SI. The AUC for egg allergy was 0.74 for egg white and 0.82 for ovomucoid in ROC analysis of HEA+ versus HEA–, and 0.72 and 0.84, respectively, in ROC analysis of REA+ versus REA– (fig. 2a), demonstrating that the parameter was higher after stimulation with ovomucoid in both ROC analyses. The cutoff value for CD203c SI in ROC analysis of HEA+ versus HEA– was 2.4 for egg white and 1.7 for ovomucoid. The sensitivity, specificity, PPV, NPV and efficiency were 73.7, 61.5, 84.8, 44.4 and 70.6%, respectively, for egg white and 80.0, 72.7, 90.3, 53.3 and 78.3%, respectively, for ovomucoid. The cutoff value for CD203c SI in ROC analysis of REA+ versus REA– was 1.7, the sensitivity, specificity, PPV, NPV and efficiency were 76.7, 62.5, 91.7, 33.3 and 74.5%, respectively, for egg white. The cutoff value was 1.6 for ovomucoid, and the sensitivity, specificity, PPV, NPV and efficiency were 82.5, 83.3, 97.1, 41.7 and 82.6%, respectively.

For milk allergy, the AUC for milk induced CD203c SI was higher than that for casein (0.84 vs. 0.67; fig. 2b). The cutoff value for CD203c SI was 1.9 for milk and 1.3 for casein. The sensitivity, specificity, PPV, NPV and efficiency were 88.9, 82.6, 85.7, 86.4 and 86.0% for milk and 66.7, 70.6, 73.7, 63.2, and 68.4% for casein, respectively.

As shown in figure 3a, for HEA, the threshold of CD203c expression for egg white and ovomucoid was ≥10 ng/ml. Eighteen of 19 patients (95%) were HEA+ when the threshold of CD203c expression for egg white was 10 ng/ml ($p < 0.01$). All of the 21 patients (100%) were HEA+ when the threshold of CD203c expression for ovomucoid was 10 ng/ml ($p < 0.01$). When diagnoses were

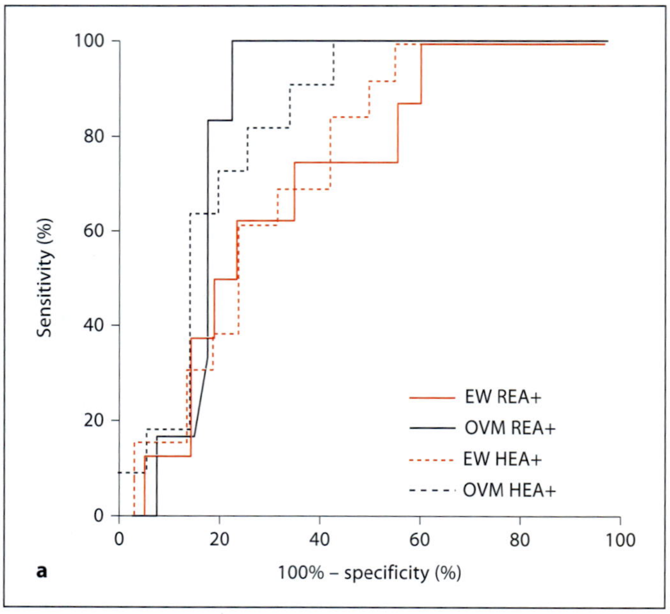

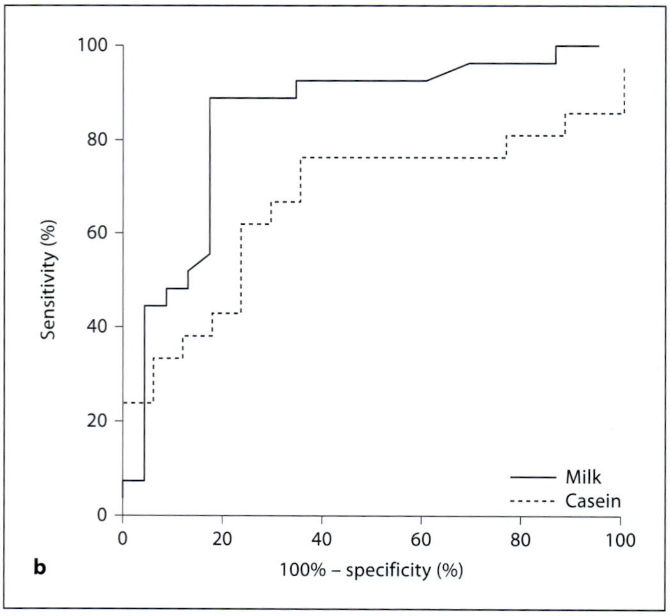

Fig. 2. ROC curves for CD203c SI induced by food antigen in patients with hen's egg allergy (**a**) and cow's milk allergy (**b**). OVM = Ovomucoid.

based on these threshold concentrations, sensitivity, specificity, PPV, NPV and efficiency were 47.4, 92.3, 94.7, 37.5 and 66.7%, respectively, for egg white and 60.0, 100.0, 100.0, 44.0 and 69.6%, respectively, for ovomucoid in HEA+ patients.

Although 18 of the 19 patients (95%) were REA+ when the threshold of CD203c expression for egg white was 10 ng/ml, no significant difference was seen between REA+ and REA– patients. All of the 30 patients (100%) were REA+ when the threshold of CD203c expression for ovomucoid was ≤1,000 ng/ml ($p < 0.01$). When diagnoses were based on these threshold concentrations, sensitivity, specificity, PPV, NPV and efficiency were 41.9, 87.5, 94.7, 21.9 and 49.0%, respectively, for egg white and 73.2, 100.0, 100.0, 31.3 and 76.1%, respectively, for ovomucoid in REA+ patients (fig. 3b).

As shown in figure 3c, 24 of the 28 patients (86%) were MA+ when the threshold of CD203c expression for milk was ≤1,000 ng/ml ($p < 0.01$). Twelve of the 16 patients (75%) were MA+ when the threshold of CD203c expression for casein was ≤1,000 ng/ml (nonsignificant). When diagnoses were based on these threshold concentrations, sensitivity, specificity, PPV, NPV and efficiency for milk were 88.9, 82.6, 85.7, 86.4 and 52.6%, respectively, and 57.1, 76.5, 75.0, 59.1 and 52.6%, respectively, for casein in MA+ patients.

Discussion

Generally, indications for OFC are individually determined considering the patient's history and antigen-specific IgE levels. However, OFC may sometimes cause severe allergic reactions. In recent years, measurement of CD203c expression on basophils has become a promising diagnostic procedure for IgE-dependent allergy.

In the present study, we demonstrated that in patients with egg allergy, the maximum CD203c expression by ovomucoid was significantly higher in the HEA+ group, and in patients with milk allergy, the maximum CD203c expression by milk was also significantly higher in the MA+ group. In a study by Ocmant et al. [17], CD203c expression was up-regulated after ovalbumin stimulation in patients with egg allergy, and CD203c SI had a sensitivity of 62.5% and a specificity of 96.5% and could be useful in the diagnosis of FA. These findings suggested that the levels of CD203c expression induced by these antigens reflect the presence of egg and milk allergies.

Regarding HEA, the AUC received from ROC analysis for ovomucoid CD203c SI was higher than for egg white (0.84 vs. 0.72, respectively). Similarly, regarding REA, the AUC received from ROC analysis for ovomucoid CD203c SI was also higher than for egg white (0.82 vs. 0.74, respectively). In addition, using the cutoff value obtained from

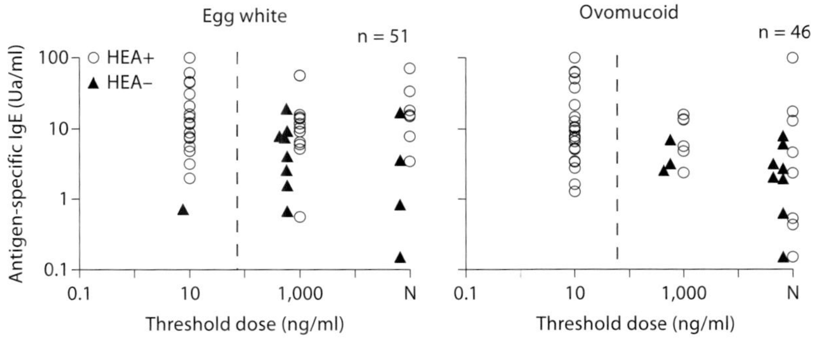

Threshold ng/ml	HEA+	HEA–	Total
≤10	18*	1	19
>10	20	12	32
Total	38	13	51

Threshold ng/ml	HEA+	HEA–	Total
≤10	21*	0	21
>10	14	11	25
Total	35	11	46

a

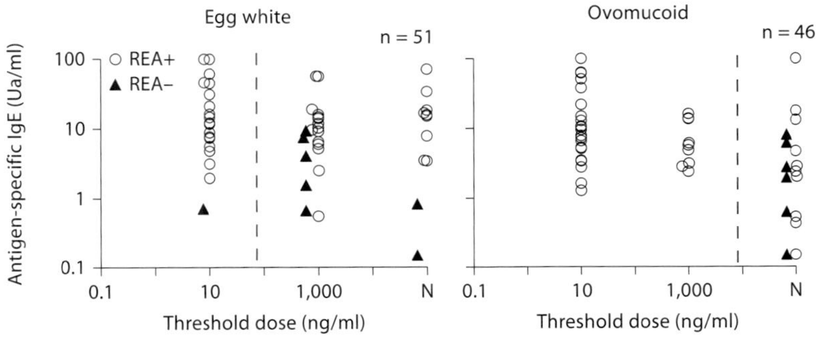

Threshold ng/ml	REA+	REA–	Total
≤10	18	1	19
>10	25	7	32
Total	43	8	51

Threshold ng/m	REA+	REA–	Total
≤1,000	30*	0	30
>1,000	10	6	16
Total	40	6	46

b

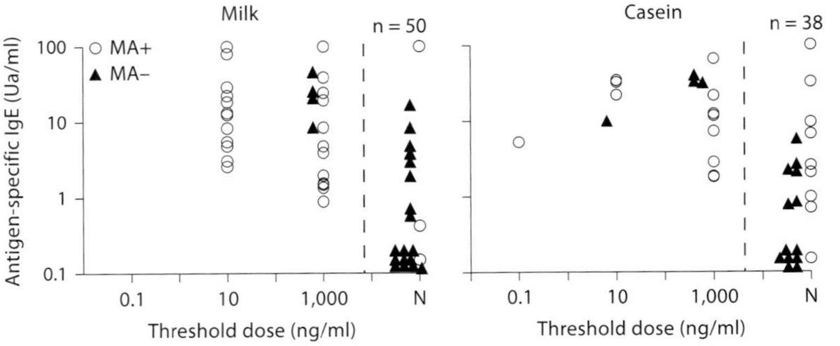

Threshold ng/ml	MA+	MA–	Total
≤1,000	24*	4	28
>1,000	3	19	22
Total	27	23	50

Threshold ng/ml	MA+	MA–	Total
≤1,000	12	4	16
>1,000	9	13	22
Total	21	17	38

c

Fig. 3. Diagnosis of FA and its relationship to antigen-specific IgE and threshold of CD203c expression. **a** Heated-egg allergy. **b** Raw-egg allergy. **c** Cow's milk allergy. * $p < 0.01$, χ^2 test. N = CD203c SI at the maximum concentration of antigen is <2.

the ROC analysis, the PPV of ovomucoid CD203c SI was higher than that for egg white in both HEA and REA. These results indicate that after stimulation with ovomucoid CD203c SI is a useful predictor of OFC-associated symptoms in egg allergy.

When the threshold of egg white-induced CD203c expression was used in the diagnosis of HEA, sensitivity, specificity and PPV were 47.4, 92.3 and 94.7%, respectively, for egg white and 60.0, 100.0 and 100.0%, respectively, for ovomucoid. When the threshold of CD203c expression was used in the diagnosis of REA, sensitivity, specificity and PPV were 41.9, 87.5 and 94.7%, respectively, for egg white and 75.0, 100.0 and 100.0%, respectively, for ovomucoid, indicating the higher PPV for CD203c expression than CD203c SI.

Antigen-specific IgE levels were reported to be instrumental in predicting OFC outcomes in children [4]. However, the outcomes of OFCs depend on the individual patient even if antigen-specific IgE levels are the same. The threshold for CD203c also depends on the individual patient even if antigen-specific IgE levels are the same. When the threshold for CD203c after stimulation by egg white or ovomucoid is 10 ng/ml, OFCs are likely to elicit allergic reactions regardless of antigen-specific IgE levels. To our knowledge, our study is the first report dealing with diagnostic analyses of the threshold for antigen-induced CD203c. On the other hand, patients with birch pollen allergy complicated with oral allergy syndrome had low concentrations and thresholds to birch pollen-induced histamine release compared to those with birch pollen allergy not complicated with oral allergy syndrome [20], suggesting that CD203c expression may be enhanced at lower concentrations in patients with allergic symptoms compared to patients without them.

Sensitivity and specificity of CD203 SI or the threshold of CD203c expression slightly differed between HEA and REA. Sensitivity and specificity after stimulation by egg white were almost similar between HEA and REA, whereas those after stimulation by ovomucoid were higher for HEA than REA. Eggs are sensitive to thermal denaturation [21], and antigenicity may depend on the heating conditions of the food tested. Ovomucoid, an egg white allergen, is rather resistant to heat [22]. Ovomucoid-specific IgE levels were high in patients with HEA [23]. This implies that patients with HEA responded to heat-resistant ovomucoid, and ovomucoid may thus be a better stimulatory allergen in the diagnosis of such patients.

The benefit of milk-induced CD203c expression on basophils in the diagnosis of milk allergy has not been documented previously. In the present study, the AUC received from ROC analysis for milk-induced CD203c SI was higher than for casein (0.84 vs. 0.67, respectively). In addition, using the cutoff value obtained from ROC analysis, sensitivity, specificity and PPV of milk-induced CD203c SI were 88.9, 82.6 and 85.7%, respectively, and those after stimulation by casein were 66.7, 70.6 and 73.7%, respectively. The PPV of milk-induced CD203c SI was higher than that for casein.

When the threshold of milk-induced CD203c expression was used in the diagnosis of milk allergy, sensitivity, specificity and PPV were 88.9, 82.6 and 85.7%, respectively. These results were similar to those obtained when the CD203c SI was used. There was no significant difference between MA+ and MA– patients using the threshold of casein-induced CD203c expression. These data indicate that using a threshold of milk-induced CD203c expression $\leq$1,000 ng/ml, OFCs are likely to elicit allergic reactions regardless of antigen-specific IgE levels.

In conclusion, OFCs are likely to elicit allergic reactions in egg or milk allergy patients when the threshold of ovomucoid-induced CD203c is 10 mg/ml or when the threshold of milk-induced CD203c is $\leq$1,000 ng/ml. Consequently, analysis of CD203c expression on basophils may be beneficial in the diagnosis of FA.

Acknowledgments

We thank all staff members who participated in this study at the Sagamihara National Hospital. This study was supported by Health and Labor Science Research Grants for the Research on Allergic Diseases and Immunology from the Ministry of Health, Labor and Welfare, Japan.

Disclosure Statement

The authors declare that no financial or other conflict of interest exists in relation to the content of this article.

References

1 Skripak JM, Matsui EC, Mudd K, Wood RA: The natural history of IgE-mediated cow's milk allergy. J Allergy Clin Immunol 2007; 120:1172–1177.
2 Sampson HA: Utility of food-specific IgE concentrations in predicting symptomatic food allergy. J Allergy Clin Immunol 2001; 107:891–896.
3 Sampson HA, Ho DG: Relationship between food-specific IgE concentrations and the risk of positive food challenges in children and adolescents. J Allergy Clin Immunol 1997; 100:444–451.

4 Komata T, Soderstrom L, Borres MP, Tachimoto H, Ebisawa M: The predictive relationship of food-specific serum IgE concentrations to challenge outcomes for egg and milk varies by patient age. J Allergy Clin Immunol 2007;119:1272–1274.
5 Lichtenstein LM, Osler AG: Studies on the mechanisms of hypersensitivity phenomena. IX. Histamine release from human leukocytes by ragweed pollen antigen. J Exp Med 1964;120:507–530.
6 Ebo DG, Sainte-Laudy J, Bridts CH, Mertens CH, Hagendorens MM, Schuerwegh AJ, De Clerck LS, Stevens WJ: Flow-assisted allergy diagnosis: current applications and future perspectives. Allergy 2006;61:1028–1039.
7 de Weck AL, Sanz ML, Gamboa PM, Aberer W, Bienvenu J, Blanca M, Demoly P, Ebo DG, Mayorga L, Monneret G, Sainte-Laudy J: Diagnostic tests based on human basophils: more potentials and perspectives than pitfalls. Int Arch Allergy Immunol 2008;146: 177–189.
8 Boumiza R, Monneret G, Forissier MF, Savoye J, Gutowski MC, Powell WS, Bienvenu J: Marked improvement of the basophil activation test by detecting CD203c instead of CD63. Clin Exp Allergy 2003;33:259–265.
9 Gober LM, Eckman JA, Sterba PM, Vasagar K, Schroeder JT, Golden DB, Saini SS: Expression of activation markers on basophils in a controlled model of anaphylaxis. J Allergy Clin Immunol 2007;119:1181–1188.
10 Binder M, Fierlbeck G, King T, Valent P, Buhring HJ: Individual hymenoptera venom compounds induce upregulation of the basophil activation marker ectonucleotide pyrophosphatase/phosphodiesterase 3 (CD203c) in sensitized patients. Int Arch Allergy Immunol 2002;129:160–168.
11 Hauswirth AW, Natter S, Ghannadan M, Majlesi Y, Schernthaner GH, Sperr WR, Buhring HJ, Valenta R, Valent P: Recombinant allergens promote expression of CD203c on basophils in sensitized individuals. J Allergy Clin Immunol 2002;110:102–109.
12 Platz IJ, Binder M, Marxer A, Lischka G, Valent P, Buhring HJ: Hymenoptera-venom-induced upregulation of the basophil activation marker ecto-nucleotide pyrophosphatase/phosphodiesterase 3 in sensitized individuals. Int Arch Allergy Immunol 2001; 126:335–342.
13 Buhring HJ, Streble A, Valent P: The basophil-specific ectoenzyme E-NNP3 (CD203c) as a marker for cell activation and allergy diagnosis. Int Arch Allergy Immunol 2004; 133:317–329.
14 Buhring HJ, Simmons PJ, Pudney M, Muller R, Jarrossay D, van Agthoven A, Willheim M, Brugger W, Valent P, Kanz L: The monoclonal antibody 97A6 defines a novel surface antigen expressed on human basophils and their multipotent and unipotent progenitors. Blood 1999;94:2343–2356.
15 Buhring HJ, Seiffert M, Giesert C, Marxer A, Kanz L, Valent P, Sano K: The basophil activation marker defined by antibody 97A6 is identical to the ectonucleotide pyrophosphatase/phosphodiesterase 3. Blood 2001;97: 3303–3305.
16 Tokuda R, Nagao M, Hiraguchi Y, Hosoki K, Matsuda T, Kouno K, Morita E, Fujisawa T: Antigen-induced expression of CD203c on basophils predicts IgE-mediated wheat allergy. Allergol Int 2009;58:193–199.
17 Ocmant A, Mulier S, Hanssens L, Goldman M, Casimir G, Mascart F, Schandene L: Basophil activation tests for the diagnosis of food allergy in children. Clin Exp Allergy 2009;39:1234–1245.
18 Ebisawa M: Food Allergy Management Guidelines 2008 by the National Food Allergy Research Group Supported by the Ministry of Health, Welfare, and Labor, 2008.
19 Ebisawa M, Akasawa A, Kunou M, Iikura Y: Establishment of diagnosis of food allergy: food challenge test by using dry powdered foods. Iryo 2000;54:79–84.
20 Kleine-Tebbe J, Galleani M, Jeep S, Pilz B, Baisch A, Kunkel G: Basophil histamine release in patients with birch pollen hypersensitivity with and without allergic symptoms to fruits. Allergy 1992;47:618–623.
21 Bernhisel-Broadbent J, Dintzis HM, Dintzis RZ, Sampson HA: Allergenicity and antigenicity of chicken egg ovomucoid (Gal d I) compared with ovalbumin (Gal d I) in children with egg allergy and in mice. J Allergy Clin Immunol 1994;93:1047–1059.
22 Urisu A, Ando H, Morita Y, Wada E, Yasaki T, Yamada K, Komada K, Torii S, Goto M, Wakamatsu T: Allergenic activity of heated and ovomucoid-depleted egg white. J Allergy Clin Immunol 1997;100:171–176.
23 Ando H, Moverare R, Kondo Y, Tsuge I, Tanaka A, Borres MP, Urisu A: Utility of ovomucoid-specific IgE concentrations in predicting symptomatic egg allergy. J Allergy Clin Immunol 2008;122:583–588.

Original Paper

International Archives of Allergy and Immunology

Int Arch Allergy Immunol 2010;152(suppl 1):62–66
DOI: 10.1159/000312127

Published online: June 4, 2010

Serum Eosinophil Cationic Protein and 27 Cytokines/Chemokines in Acute Exacerbation of Childhood Asthma

Masahiko Kato[a] Yoshiyuki Yamada[a] Kenichi Maruyama[b] Yasuhide Hayashi[c]

Departments of [a]Allergy and Immunology, [b]Internal Medicine, and [c]Hematology and Oncology, Gunma Children's Medical Center, Shibukawa, Japan

Key Words

Asthma · Childhood asthma · Corticosteroids · Eosinophil cationic protein · Eosinophils · IL-5

Abstract

Background: Little information is available on eosinophil activation and cytokine/chemokine responses in childhood asthma, thus we examined serum eosinophil cationic protein (ECP) and 27 types of cytokines/chemokines in acute exacerbation of asthma (acute asthma) and stable asthma. ***Methods:*** We determined peripheral eosinophil count, and the serum levels of ECP and 27 types of cytokines/chemokines (IL-1β, IL-1ra, IL-2, -4, -5, -6, -7, -8, -9, -10, -12, -13, -15 and -17, IFN-γ, IP-10, TNF-α, GM-CSF, G-CSF, MCP-1, MIP-1α and -1β, eotaxin, RANTES, PDGF-bb, FGF basic and VEGF) using a multiplex bead-based assay in 85 acute and 79 stable asthma patients, and 14 controls. We also examined the effects of systemic corticosteroids on these responses in acute asthma. ***Results:*** The serum levels of ECP, IL-5, -6, -8 and -10, G-CSF, MCP-1, IL-1ra and IP-10 were significantly elevated in acute compared with stable asthma. Similarly, serum levels of ECP, IL-5 and IP-10 were significantly higher in acute asthma than in controls. Furthermore, in the acute phase, elevated serum levels of ECP, IL-5, IL-6, IL-1ra and IP-10, but not IL-8, IL-10, G-CSF and MCP-1 were significantly reduced after treatments that included systemic corticosteroids. ***Conclusion:*** Eosinophil activation could be induced by acute exacerbation of childhood asthma.

Introduction

Eosinophils are important effector cells in host defense against parasites and in allergic diseases such as bronchial asthma. In allergic inflammation, mediators released from epithelial or inflammatory cells induce the migration of eosinophils from the blood into the affected tissues. After migration, eosinophils are activated by appropriate stimuli resulting in the release of inflammatory mediators that include arachidonic acid metabolites, such as platelet-activating factor or cystenyl leukotrienes, oxygen radicals, cytokines/chemokines and toxic cationic granule proteins, such as major basic protein, eosinophil peroxidase, eosinophil cationic protein (ECP) and eosinophil-derived neurotoxin [1, 2]. Evidence suggests that eosinophils and their product, ECP, can serve as markers of disease activity in asthma [3]. On the other hand, several cytokines/chemokines are elevated in acute exacerbation of childhood asthma [4, 5].

KARGER

Fax +41 61 306 12 34
E-Mail karger@karger.ch
www.karger.com

1018–2438/10/1525–0062$26.00/0

Accessible online at:
www.karger.com/iaa

Correspondence to: Dr. Masahiko Kato
Department of Allergy and Immunology
Gunma Children's Medical Center
779 Shimohakoda, Hokkitsu-machi, Shibukawa, Gunma 377-8577 (Japan)
Tel. +81 279 52 3551, Fax +81 279 52 2045, E-Mail mkato@gcmc.pref.gunma.jp

The purpose of this study was to investigate changes in the serum levels of ECP and several cytokines and chemokines in acute exacerbation of childhood asthma, and to evaluate eosinophil activation in children with bronchial asthma.

Patients and Methods

Patients

The subjects who visited and/or were hospitalized with acute respiratory symptoms (acute asthma: 54 males and 31 females; mean age, 3.9 years), or who visited for regular physical examinations and treatment (stable asthma: 48 males and 31 females; mean age, 5.0 years) at the Gunma Children's Medical Center between November 1, 2003, and October 31, 2006, were enrolled in this study. All recruited patients had a history of three or more separate episodes of recurrent wheezing and documented evidence of wheezing by auscultation. The diagnosis of asthma and its severity in patients with acute exacerbations (mild attack, 4; moderate attack, 79, and severe attack, 2) were defined according to the guidelines of the Japanese Society of Pediatric Allergy and Clinical Immunology [6]. Acute asthma was diagnosed by the emergency department physician based on the presence of wheezing and increased difficulty of breathing. Briefly, a mild attack was defined as mild wheezing, with stable disease and no dyspnea, and an $S_pO_2 \geq 96\%$; a moderate attack was defined as wheezing with dyspnea, apparent retraction and an S_pO_2 from 92 to 95%, and a severe attack was defined as more severe wheezing and dyspnea, and an $S_pO_2 \leq 91\%$. Patients with mild-moderate attacks were treated with intravenous infusion, and salbutamol and disodium cromoglycate inhalation (three times/day). Patients who experienced a severe attack were treated with isoproterenol inhalation instead of salbutamol. When S_pO_2 was $\leq 95\%$, oxygen therapy was started. Most patients with acute asthma were treated with intravenous prednisolone for 3–5 days.

The patients with acute asthma had a history of a cold prior to exacerbation. We excluded children with obvious bacterial infections, congenital heart diseases, chronic lung diseases, children who presented with a foreign body or had signs of severe infection, and those who were immunosuppressed, as these complications could interfere with the assessment of asthma-related outcome measures. Stable asthma was defined as physician-diagnosed asthma which was stable (no wheezing) at the time of examination and for at least 3 months prior to the examination. Previous treatment consisted of short-acting β_2-agonists and/or long-term treatment for asthma control without systemic corticosteroids. The control group included 14 healthy children (9 males and 5 females; mean age, 3.6 years) with no symptoms of wheezing at the time of examination. Exclusion criteria for the controls were immunosuppression, the presence of other respiratory tract symptoms or a history of previous wheezing and asthma. We attempted to match asthma patients and controls for age and sex. This study was approved by the Ethics Committee of the Gunma Children's Medical Center. Informed consent was obtained from the parents, and assent was obtained from the children when they were old enough (usually >9 years old).

Serum ECP and Cytokines/Chemokines

We determined peripheral eosinophil count and the serum levels of ECP and 27 types of cytokines/chemokines, interleukin (IL)-1β, IL-1 receptor antagonist (IL-1ra), IL-2, -4, -5, -6, -7, -8, -9, -10, -12, -13, -15 and -17, interferon (IFN)-γ, IFN-γ-induced protein (IP)-10, tumor necrosis factor (TNF)-α, granulocyte-macrophage (GM) colony-stimulating factor (CSF), granulocyte CSF (G-CSF), monocyte chemoattractant protein (MCP)-1, macrophage inflammatory protein (MIP)-1α and -1β, eotaxin, RANTES (regulated on activation, normal T cell expressed and secreted), platelet-derived growth factor-bb, basic fibroblast growth factor and vascular endothelial growth factor, from 85 acute and 79 stable asthma patients who were not on systemic corticosteroids at the time of examination, and from 14 controls. To analyze the effects of treatment including systemic corticosteroids, these parameters were measured both at the time of admission and at the time when wheezing disappeared (mean days after admission = 7.3), and the levels before and after treatment were compared for each factor in 56 acute asthmatic patients. ECP content in serum was measured with a fluoroenzyme immunoassay kit (Pharmacia, Uppsala, Sweden). Serum cytokines/chemokines were determined by a multicytokine detection system (Bio-Rad, Hercules, Calif., USA), following the manufacturer's instructions, using a Luminex System (Luminex, Austin, Tex., USA) and then quantified using Bio-Plex software (Bio-Rad).

Statistical Analysis

Data were expressed as means ± SEM. Paired and unpaired data were analyzed by Wilcoxon and Mann-Whitney U test, respectively. A statistically significant difference was defined as $p < 0.05$ (two-tailed). All analyses were performed with a statistical software package (SPSS for Windows, version 12.0; SPSS Japan, Tokyo, Japan).

Results

Serum ECP and Cytokines/Chemokines

The serum levels of ECP, IL-5, -6, -8 and -10, G-CSF, IL-1ra, MCP-1 and IP-10 were significantly elevated in acute compared with stable asthma (table 1). By contrast, eosinophil counts were slightly but significantly decreased in acute asthma compared with stable asthma. Similarly, serum levels of ECP, IL-5 and IP-10 were significantly higher in acute asthma compared with controls. Furthermore, only ECP was significantly elevated in stable asthma compared with controls. No significant difference was found between mild, moderate and severe attacks in acute asthma for any parameter (data not shown). Finally, in the acute phase, elevated serum levels of ECP, IL-5, IL-6, IL-1ra and IP-10 were significantly reduced after treatment with systemic corticosteroids (fig. 1). However, treatment did not significantly affect elevated serum levels of IL-8, IL-10, G-CSF and MCP-1 in the acute phase (data not shown).

Table 1. Elevated ECP and cytokines/chemokines in patients with acute compared with stable asthma or controls

	Acute asthma (n = 85)	Stable asthma (n = 79)	Control (n = 14)
Eosinophils	250 (0–2,846)	336 (0–1,386)	204 (0–1,976)
ECP	15.8 (3.0–109.0)$^{a, d}$	12.6 (2.6–70.9)^{d}	7.3 (3.2–80.6)
IL-1β	6.27 (0.01–52.71)	7.09 (0.24–57.72)	7.72 (2.18–31.04)
IL-1ra	406.26 (45.18–4,556.18)^{b}	201.07 (46.49–3,195.79)	213.08 (100.63–1,253.91)
IL-2	6.86 (0.43–248.75)	8.63 (0.60–232.71)	8.87 (3.57–12.01)
IL-4	15.01 (1.62–151.46)	16.18 (0.96–84.63)	15.54 (2.04–73.31)
IL-5	4.97 (0.07–118.44)$^{b, c}$	2.23 (0.07–19.33)	3.10 (0.02–7.64)
IL-6	80.49 (12.49–794.13)^{b}	55.44 (1.10–1,138.54)	59.86 (14.12–238.48)
IL-7	15.34 (1.46–42.8)	14.35 (0.83–29.21)	16.87 (0.83–27.14)
IL-8	12.84 (0.21–171.26)^{b}	6.19 (0.36–27.54)	9.38 (0.36–38.39)
IL-9	58.75 (5.44–2,036.17)	51.87 (20.30–731.00)	39.00 (29.37–72.90)
IL-10	16.58 (0.13–145.43)^{b}	3.74 (0.13–54.52)	19.82 (0.35–64.32)
IL-12	5.60 (0.54–91.06)	6.77 (0.94–256.53)	6.99 (0.29–52.25)
IL-13	3.09 (0.07–26.26)	3.28 (0.12–9.69)	3.62 (1.70–4.63)
IL-15	10.08 (1.20–71.27)	8.77 (1.23–201.70)	16.99 (3.38–90.08)
IL-17	7.35 (0.09–51.07)	8.70 (0.41–43.58)	0.06 (0.06–0.06)
IFN-γ	129.82 (3.53–529.57)	134.87 (0.263–401.78)	149.47 (44.77–1,061.34)
IP-10	1,395.52 (158.06–23,554.11)$^{b, d}$	439.48 (140.80–1,325.22)	541.85 (330.86–1,981.86)
TNF-α	19.51 (0.07–682.83)	32.54 (0.25–97.92)	30.11 (0.25–392.13)
GM-CSF	33.82 (0.20–962.04)	21.80 (2.33–327.07)	22.23 (0.56–71.99)
G-CSF	43.88 (2.24–1,341.93)^{a}	34.71 (0.24–275.39)	38.03 (19.42–129.62)
MCP-1	54.96 (13.01–254.60)^{a}	46.21 (5.50–102.64)	62.98 (30.23–96.89)
MIP-1α	12.26 (1.47–46.77)	12.61 (4.72–25.20)	12.95 (10.60–14.79)
MIP-1β	80.72 (6.00–275.91)	99.40 (18.37–304.12)	116.91 (15.26–168.02)
Eotaxin	80.95 (35.48–440.78)	97.61 (18.30–949.34)	112.81(69.83–577.43)
RANTES	5,339.63 (2,146.85–114,340.39)	9,089.88 (4,994.69–25,210.45)	5,831.70 (4,632.50–7,030.89)
PDGF-bb	7,273.09 (433.33–19,544.26)	7,730.38 (3,657.11–15,311.06)	6,540.45 (2,622.59–12,493.89)
FGF-basic	68.63 (15.39–471.64)	96.76 (24.72–280.66)	71.97 (35.20–156.77)
VEGF	115.74 (5.22–729.05)	107.33 (20.14–1,287.23)	65.81 (18.13–270.06)

Medians (ranges), Mann-Whitney U test, ^{a} $p < 0.05$; ^{b} $p < 0.001$, vs. stable asthma; ^{c} $p < 0.05$; ^{d} $p < 0.01$, vs. control. PDGF-bb = Platelet-derived growth factor-bb; FGF = fibroblast growth factor; VEGF = vascular endothelial growth factor. Eosinophils: n/mm^3; ECP: ng/ml, and cytokines/chemokines: pg/ml.

Discussion

Although previous reports showed serum ECP [7–10] and serum or plasma cytokine/chemokine production [7, 10–19] in acute exacerbations of asthma, this is the first report to show the profiles of ECP and 27 cytokines/chemokines in serum samples of patients with acute and stable asthma, and in controls. In this study, serum ECP was significantly elevated in acute asthma compared with stable asthma and controls. Similarly, in previous reports, serum levels of ECP were significantly higher in children with acute asthma than in those with stable asthma and controls [7, 8]. These results suggest that acute exacerbation of asthma might enhance eosinophil activity, e.g. degranulation.

Oymar et al. [7] also reported that the serum level of IL-5 was significantly elevated in children with acute asthma. In an analysis of the correlation between each factor using data from patients with acute asthma, a significant association was found between peripheral blood eosinophil count and serum ECP ($r = 0.541$, $p < 0.0001$), and between ECP and IL-5 ($r = 0.310$, $p = 0.0015$). These results suggest that eosinophil activation during acute asthma is mediated at least in part by IL-5.

Th2 cytokines are thought to mediate most of the allergic inflammatory responses associated with atopic asthma. However, the Th1-related chemokine IP-10/CXCL10 was the predominant chemokine measured during human allergic pulmonary late-phase reactions [20]. In our study, the serum level of IP-10 was also signifi-

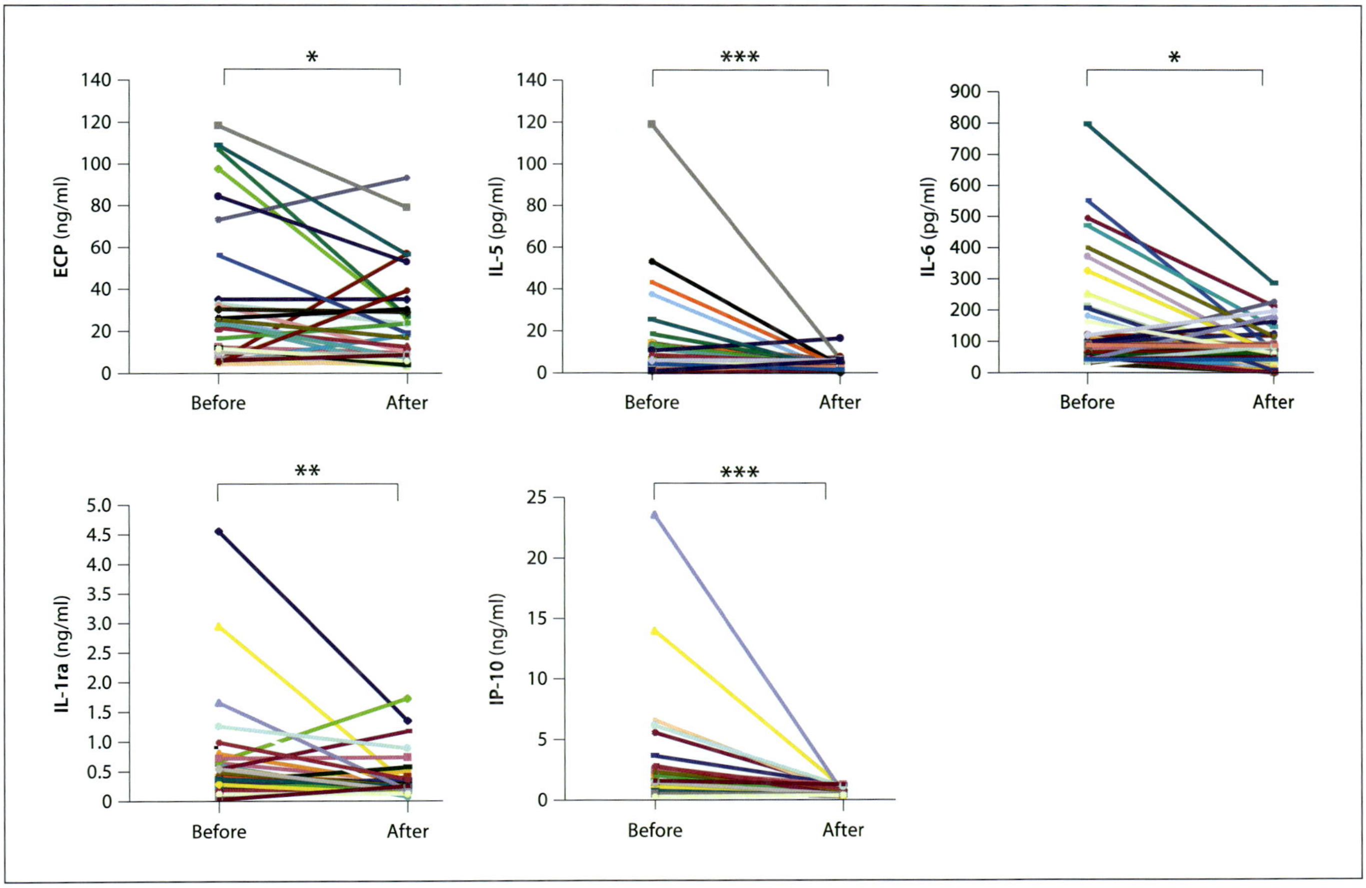

Fig. 1. Effect of treatment that included systemic corticosteroids on elevated serum levels of ECP and cytokines/chemokines in acute asthma. In the acute phase, elevated serum levels of ECP, IL-5, IL-6, IL-1ra and IP-10 were significantly decreased after treatment. Differently colored lines show the values for each subject. * $p < 0.05$; ** $p < 0.01$; *** $p < 0.001$, before vs. after treatment; Wilcoxon test.

cantly higher in acute asthma than in stable asthma and controls. In similar reports, serum or plasma levels of IP-10 were increased in acute asthma, specifically in cases of rhinovirus infection [14, 15], suggesting that IP-10 is a novel marker of acute exacerbation of asthma induced by rhinoviruses. However, these studies failed to clarify the viral pathogen. IL-1ra is a potent anti-inflammatory cytokine [21]. Previously, serum levels of soluble TNF-receptor I and II, and IL-1ra obtained during bronchial asthma attacks were higher than those from patients in stable condition [16]. This report and our results indicate that higher serum levels of IL-1ra may reflect the up-regulation of IL-1ra production in acute asthma, and that IL-1ra may contribute to TNF-α- and IL-1-mediated production of IL-1ra per se in acute asthma.

IL-8 and G-CSF are major cytokines in the recruitment of neutrophils to the inflammatory area [22]. Tang and Chen [12] reported that the serum level of IL-8 was significantly higher in children with acute asthma and in stable asthmatics than in control subjects. In contrast to our results, the difference between acute and stable asthmatics was not significant, indicating that serum IL-8 is a poor indicator of disease activity in asthma.

Corticosteroid therapy is one of the most effective treatments for asthma. However, evidence suggests that treatment with inhaled corticosteroids does not improve airway inflammation induced by rhinovirus infection [23]. On the other hand, oral glucocorticoids improve lung function and decrease serum IL-6, soluble ICAM-1 and ECP levels [10]. In this study, treatment comprising systemic corticosteroids resulted in decreases in serum levels of ECP, IL-5, IL-6, IL-1ra and IP-10, but not IL-8, IL-10, G-CSF and MCP-1. In previous studies, systemic corticosteroid treatment of children with asthma significantly reduced serum concentrations of ECP [24–26], IL-5 [26] and IP-10 [12]. Furthermore, systemic corticosteroids significantly reduced both IL-5 gene expression and serum levels of ECP in acute compared with stable asthma [27]. These results suggest that systemic corticosteroids might reduce eosinophil activation via IL-5 production. However, since this investigation was not a case-control study of systemic corticosteroids, a study designed to discover the exact effects of systemic corticosteroids is needed.

Further investigation into the mechanisms behind the association between asthma exacerbations and eosinophil activation is required.

Acknowledgments

This study was supported, in part, by grants-in-aid for scientific research (Nos. 18591208 and 20591267) from the Ministry of Education, Culture, Sports, Sciences and Technology, the Ministry of Environment and Gunma Prefecture (Japan). We thank Dr. Makoto Todokoro and other doctors who work for the Gunma Children's Medical Center for collecting the samples.

Disclosure Statement

The authors declare that no financial or other conflict of interest exists in relation to the content of this article.

References

1 Gleich GJ: Mechanisms of eosinophil-associated inflammation. J Allergy Clin Immunol 2000;105:651–663.

2 Kato M, Suzuki M, Hayashi Y, Kimura H: Role of eosinophils and their clinical significance in allergic inflammation. Expert Rev Clin Immunol 2006;2:121–133.

3 Ferguson AC, Vaughan R, Brown H, Curtis C: Evaluation of serum eosinophilic cationic protein as a marker of disease activity in chronic asthma. J Allergy Clin Immunol 1995;95:23–28.

4 Cohn L, Elias JA, Chupp GL: Asthma: mechanisms of disease persistence and progression. Annu Rev Immunol 2004;22:789–815.

5 Palmqvist C, Wardlaw AJ, Bradding P: Chemokines and their receptors as potential targets for the treatment of asthma. Br J Pharmacol 2007;151:725–736.

6 Nishimuta T, Nishima S, Morikawa A (eds): Japanese Pediatric Society: Japanese Pediatric Guidelines for the Treatment and Management of Asthma 2008 (in Japanese). Tokyo, Kyowakikaku, 2008, pp 14–16.

7 Oymar K, Elsayed S, Bjerknes R: Serum eosinophil cationic protein and interleukin-5 in children with bronchial asthma and acute bronchiolitis. Pediatr Allergy Immunol 1996;7:180–186.

8 Tang RB, Chen SJ: Serum levels of eosinophil cationic protein and eosinophils in asthmatic children during a course of prednisolone therapy. Pediatr Pulmonol 2001;31:121–125.

9 Koh YY, Kang H, Kim CK: Ratio of serum eosinophil cationic protein/blood eosinophil counts in children with asthma: comparison between acute exacerbation and clinical remission. Allergy Asthma Proc 2003;24:269–274.

10 Yasuda H, Suzuki T, Zayasu K, Ishizuka S, Kubo H, Sasaki T, Nishimura H, Sekizawa K, Yamaya M: Inflammatory and bronchospastic factors in asthma exacerbations caused by upper respiratory tract infections. Tohoku J Exp Med 2005;207:109–118.

11 Tang RB, Chen SJ: Soluble interleukin-2 receptor and interleukin-4 in sera of asthmatic children before and after a prednisolone course. Ann Allergy Asthma Immunol 2001; 86:314–317.

12 Tang RB, Chen SJ: Evaluation of serum interleukin-8 as a marker of disease activity in acute asthma in children. J Asthma 2000;37: 409–413.

13 Tsai TC, Lu JH, Chen SJ, Tang RB: Soluble interleukin-10 and transforming growth factor-β in children with acute exacerbation of allergic asthma. J Asthma 2009;46:21–24.

14 Wark PA, Bucchieri F, Johnston SL, Gibson PG, Hamilton L, Mimica J, Zummo G, Holgate ST, Attia J, Thakkinstian A, Davies DE: IFN-γ-induced protein 10 is a novel biomarker of rhinovirus-induced asthma exacerbations. J Allergy Clin Immunol 2007;120: 586–593.

15 Lai ST, Hung CH, Hua YM, Hsu SH, Jong YJ, Suen JL: T-helper 1-related chemokines in the exacerbation of childhood asthma. Pediatr Int 2008;50:99–102.

16 Yoshida S, Hashimoto S, Nakayama T, Kobayashi T, Koizumi A, Horie T: Elevation of serum soluble tumour necrosis factor (TNF) receptor and IL-1 receptor antagonist levels in bronchial asthma. Clin Exp Immunol 1996;106:73–78.

17 Lilly CM, Woodruff PG, Camargo CA Jr, Nakamura H, Drazen JM, Nadel ES, Hanrahan JP: Elevated plasma eotaxin levels in patients with acute asthma. J Allergy Clin Immunol 1999;104:786–790.

18 Chan CK, Kuo ML, Yeh KW, Ou LS, Chen LC, Yao TC, Huang JL: Sequential evaluation of serum monocyte chemotactic protein 1 among asymptomatic state and acute exacerbation and remission of asthma in children. J Asthma 2009;46:225–228.

19 Kalayci O, Sonna LA, Woodruff PG, Camargo CA Jr, Luster AD, Lilly CM: Monocyte chemotactic protein-4 (MCP-4; CCL-13): a biomarker of asthma. J Asthma 2004;41:27–33.

20 Bochner BS, Hudson SA, Xiao HQ, Liu MC: Release of both CCR4-active and CXCR3-active chemokines during human allergic pulmonary late-phase reactions. J Allergy Clin Immunol 2003;112:930–934.

21 Rosenwasser LJ: Biologic activities of IL-1 and its role in human disease. J Allergy Clin Immunol 1998;102:344–350.

22 Sampson AP: The role of eosinophils and neutrophils in inflammation. Clin Exp Allergy 2000;30(suppl 1):22–27.

23 Grünberg K, Sharon RF, Sont JK, In 't Veen JC, Van Schadewijk WA, De Klerk EP, Dick CR, Van Krieken JH, Sterk PJ: Rhinovirus-induced airway inflammation in asthma: effect of treatment with inhaled corticosteroids before and during experimental infection. Am J Respir Crit Care Med 2001; 164:1816–1822.

24 Sorkness C, McGill K, Busse WW: Evaluation of serum eosinophil cationic protein as a predictive marker for asthma exacerbation in patients with persistent disease. Clin Exp Allergy 2002;32:1355–1359.

25 Marouf R, Khadadah ME, Onadeko BO, Mustafa HT, Khamis A, Ezeamuzie CE, Sugathan TN: The effect of corticosteroid therapy on blood eosinophils and eosinophilic cationic protein in patients with acute and chronic asthma. J Asthma 1999;36:555–564.

26 Sahid El-Radhi A, Hogg CL, Bungre JK, Bush A, Corrigan CJ: Effect of oral glucocorticoid treatment on serum inflammatory markers in acute asthma. Arch Dis Child 2000;83: 158–162.

27 Lai CK, Ho AS, Chan CH, Tang J, Leung JC, Lai KN: Interleukin-5 messenger RNA expression in peripheral blood CD4+ cells in asthma. J Allergy Clin Immunol 1996;97: 1320–1328.

International Archives of
Allergy and Immunology

Original Paper

Int Arch Allergy Immunol 2010;152(suppl 1):67–74
DOI: 10.1159/000312128

Published online: June 4, 2010

Strain-Specific Phenotypes of Airway Inflammation and Bronchial Hyperresponsiveness Induced by Epicutaneous Allergen Sensitization in BALB/c and C57BL/6 Mice

Motohiro Kodama[a] Koichiro Asano[a] Tsuyoshi Oguma[a] Shizuko Kagawa[a] Katsuyoshi Tomomatsu[a] Misa Wakaki[a] Takahisa Takihara[a] Soichiro Ueda[a] Nao Ohmori[a] Hiromi Ogura[a] Jun Miyata[a] Kyuto Tanaka[a] Nobufumi Kamiishi[a] Koichi Fukunaga[a] Koichi Sayama[a] Eiji Ikeda[b] Taku Miyasho[c] Akitoshi Ishizaka[a]

[a]Division of Pulmonary Medicine, Department of Medicine, and [b]Department of Pathology, Keio University School of Medicine, Tokyo, and [c]Laboratory of Veterinary Biochemistry, Rakuno Gakuen University, Ebetsu, Japan

Key Words

Allergic airway inflammation · Asthma model · Bronchial responsiveness · C57BL/6 · Epicutaneous sensitization · Skin barrier dysfunction

Abstract

Background: Allergen sensitization through a disrupted skin barrier appears to play a prominent role in the development of atopic diseases, including allergic asthma. The role of the genetic background in immunological and physiological phenotypes induced by epicutaneous sensitization is undetermined. ***Methods:*** BALB/c and C57BL/6 mice were sensitized either epicutaneously by patch application of ovalbumin (OVA) or systemically by intraperitoneal injection of OVA with alum before exposure to aerosolized OVA. The concentrations of OVA-specific immunoglobulin in serum and cytokines in bronchoalveolar lavage fluid (BALF) were measured by enzyme-linked immunosorbent assay. The severity of airway inflammation was evaluated by cell counts in BALF, and bronchial responsiveness to methacholine was measured by the flexiVent system. ***Results:*** The production of OVA-specific IgG1 and IgE was greater in the epicutaneously sensitized BALB/c than C57BL/6 mice. In contrast, both eosinophilic airway inflammation and bronchial responsiveness to methacholine were more prominent in the C57BL/6 than in the BALB/c mice. The concentrations of interleukin-4 increased significantly in the BALF from C57BL/6 mice only. No between-strain differences were observed after intraperitoneal sensitization. ***Conclusions:*** The C57BL/6 mouse is a more appropriate model than the BALB/c mouse to study the relationship between skin barrier dysfunction and the pathogenesis of allergic asthma.

Introduction

Epidemiological observations suggest that epicutaneous sensitization is an important route of immunization to aeroallergens, such as house dust mites, predisposing to atopic dermatitis and other atopic diseases, including asthma and allergic rhinitis [1, 2]. A genetic deficiency in filaggrin, an essential molecule that maintains the cuta-

KARGER

Fax +41 61 306 12 34
E-Mail karger@karger.ch
www.karger.com

1018–2438/10/1525–0067$26.00/0

Accessible online at:
www.karger.com/iaa

Correspondence to: Dr. Koichiro Asano
Division of Pulmonary Medicine, Department of Medicine
Keio University School of Medicine
35 Shinanomachi, Shinjuku-ku, Tokyo 160-8582 (Japan)
Tel. +81 3 3353 1211, Fax +81 3 3353 2502, E-Mail ko-asano@qa2.so-net.ne.jp

neous barrier function, is present in a large proportion of patients susceptible to atopic dermatitis with or without asthma [3–5]. The role of the skin in the first-line defense against allergens has also been confirmed in experimental models of allergic dermatitis [6], rhinitis [7], asthma [8, 9] and eosinophilic esophagitis [10]. Epicutaneous sensitization with a protein antigen such as ovalbumin (OVA) followed by local exposure of the airways to the same antigen induces a predominant Th2 response with abundant production of IgE as well as eosinophilic inflammation. The effect of differences in the genetic background among inbred mouse strains on immunological and physiological phenotypes according to the route of sensitization has not been determined yet. The purpose of our study was to examine (a) the production of antigen-specific immunoglobulin, (b) the severity of airway inflammation, (c) bronchial responsiveness and (d) cytokine production in the commonly used BALB/c and C57BL/6 mouse models of allergic asthma induced by intraperitoneal versus epicutaneous sensitization.

Methods

Animal Preparations

Specific pathogen- and virus antibody-free, 6-week-old, male BALB/cAnNCrlCrlj (BALB/c) and C57BL/6J (C57BL/6) mice, weighing 25–30 g, were purchased from Charles River Laboratories, Yokohama, Japan. All animals were housed at the facility in bioBubble® barrier units (bioBubble, Fort Collins, Colo., USA) under positive pressure. The experimental protocol was reviewed and approved by the Laboratory Animal Care and Use Committee of Keio University School of Medicine.

Allergen Sensitization and Exposure

Epicutaneous sensitization was achieved with 40 μl of 4 mg/ml grade V OVA (Sigma, St. Louis, Mo., USA) in phosphate-buffered saline (PBS), or PBS alone, placed on the disk of a Finn chamber® (SmartPractice®, Phoenix, Ariz., USA). For each course of immunization, freshly prepared patches were applied to a shaved dorsal area of the mice on days 1, 8 and 15, and removed 3 days after their application. Separate groups of mice were immunized for 1 and 2 weeks, respectively, to study the relationship between the degree of sensitization and outcomes. Intraperitoneal sensitization was achieved by injections of 15 μg of OVA in alum solution (Imject®Alum, Pierce, Rockford, Ill., USA) on days 1, 8 and 15. The aerosol challenge was carried out in a dedicated chamber with 2% (w/v) OVA diluted in PBS for 20 min on days 21–24.

Bronchial Responsiveness to Methacholine

The bronchial responsiveness to methacholine (Sigma) was measured 24 h after the challenge with aerosolized OVA. The trachea was cannulated with an 18-gauge tube under anesthesia with 100 mg/kg of ketamine and 10 mg/kg of xylazine, i.p., and the animals were quasi-sinusoidally ventilated at 180 breaths/min, with a computer-controlled, small animal ventilator (flexiVent; SCIREQ, Montreal, Que., Canada), with a tidal volume of 10 ml/kg, against an artificial positive end-expiratory pressure of 3 cm H_2O. Before the measurement of airway resistance, the lungs were inflated 3 times to total capacity to standardize the volume history among animals. Resistance was measured using a 3-Hz sinusoidal piston volume movement of 10 ml/kg. The pressure-volume and flow data were fit to a single-compartment model to derive the measurements of airway resistance. Freshly prepared methacholine in PBS was delivered through an inline nebulizer in doses of 0, 3.125, 6.25, 12.5, 25.0 and 50.0 mg/ml. The direct delivery of methacholine to the lung was timed with inspiration. After each methacholine challenge, airway resistance was assessed every 15 s during tidal breathing, and the 4th measurement was used as the bronchoconstrictor response to each individual methacholine dose.

Bronchoalveolar Lavage

The mice were sacrificed by an overdose of intravenous pentobarbital, 24 h after the aerosolized OVA challenge. The trachea was cannulated and the lungs were lavaged twice with 0.7 ml of ice-cold PBS with 0.6 mM EDTA. The total number of cells in bronchoalveolar lavage fluid (BALF) was counted using a hemocytometer, and a differential cell count of 200 cells was determined on Diff-Quik-stained cytospin slides (Baxter Scientific Products, McGraw Park, Ill., USA) prepared with Auto Smear CF12D (Sakura Finetek, Tokyo, Japan).

The concentrations of interleukin (IL)-4, IL-5, IL-12 p70, IL-13, IL-17 and interferon (IFN)-γ in BALF were measured using a Bio-Plex suspension array system (Bio-Rad Laboratories, Hercules, Calif., USA) according to the manufacturer's instructions. Lower detection limits were 0.29 pg/ml for IL-4, 0.17 pg/ml for IL-5, 0.35 pg/ml for IL-12 p70, 4.43 pg/ml for IL-13, 0.31 pg/ml for IL-17 and 0.27 pg/ml for IFN-γ.

Measurement of Serum OVA-Specific IgG1 and IgE Antibodies

Whole blood was collected from the inferior vena cava on day 25, 24 h after the aerosolized OVA challenge. The protein concentration in serum was measured with the Bradford method, before dilution of the samples to 1 mg protein/ml. The concentrations of OVA-specific IgG1 and IgE antibodies in serum were measured with commercially available enzyme-linked immunosorbent assay kits (AKRIE-040 and -030, Shibayagi, Gunma, Japan). Briefly, 50 μl of the diluted samples (50 μg of protein) were applied in duplicate on 96-well plates coated with antibody to capture OVA-specific antibodies, incubated for 1 h at room temperature and washed with 0.05% PBS-Tween 20. One-step detection was obtained by incubation with biotinylated anti-IgG1 or IgE mixed with streptavidin-conjugated horseradish peroxidase for 1 h at room temperature. The plates were washed and developed with TMB substrate for 30 min. The reaction was stopped by adding 1 M H_2SO_4, immediately before reading the optical density at 450 nm. Lower detection limits were 1.88 mU/ml for IgG1 and 1.88 U/ml for IgE.

Statistical Analyses

The data are presented as means ± SEM. The numbers of leukocytes in BALF, serum Ig concentrations and concentrations of cytokines in BALF were compared using the Kruskal-Wallis test, followed by the Bonferroni/Dunn procedure as a post hoc test.

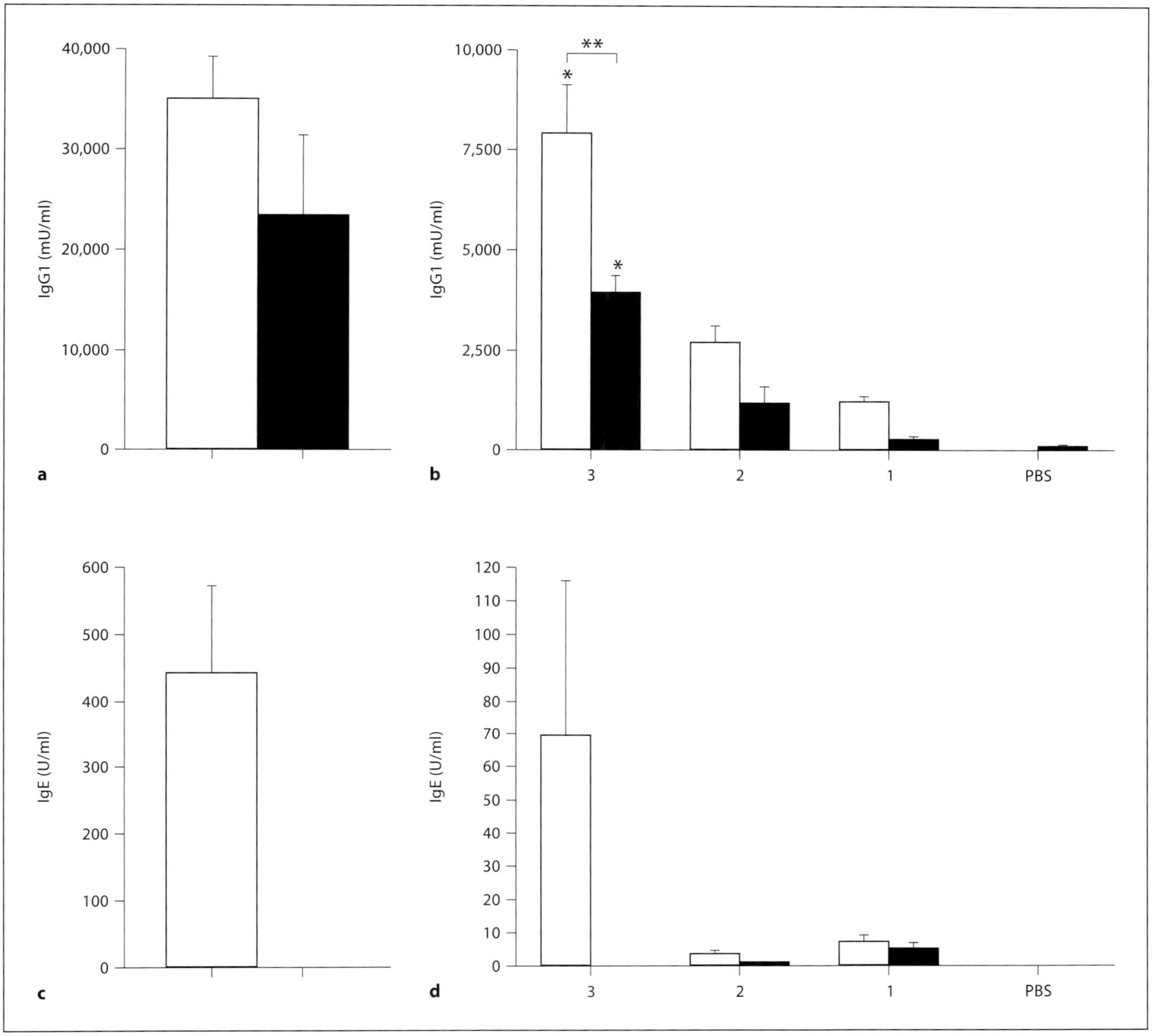

Fig. 1. Serum concentrations of OVA-specific IgG1 (**a**, **b**) and IgE (**c**, **d**). BALB/c mice (□) and C57BL/6 mice (■) were sensitized intraperitoneally to OVA with the adjuvant, alum (**a**, **c**) or epicutaneously (1–3 times) without adjuvant (**b**, **d**) for 3 weeks. Some mice were treated with skin patches containing PBS alone (PBS). Means ± SEM. n = 4–6. * $p < 0.005$ vs. animals sensitized epicutaneously with PBS, ** $p < 0.05$ between strains.

Differences between mouse strains were analyzed using the Mann-Whitney U test. Bronchial responsiveness to methacholine was curve fitted, using a one-site binding model [$y = ax/(b + x)$], and analyzed with two-way repeated-measures analysis of variance. The data were analyzed using GraphPad Prism 4.0c (GraphPad Software, San Diego, Calif., USA) and StatView 5.0 (SAS Institute, Cary, N.C., USA). A p value < 0.05 was considered statistically significant.

Results

Intraperitoneal injection of OVA with alum induced the production of allergen-specific IgG1 in both BALB/c and C57BL/6 mice (n = 4–6). No difference in serum IgG1 concentrations was observed between the strains (fig. 1a). OVA-specific IgG1 was also produced in animals sensi-

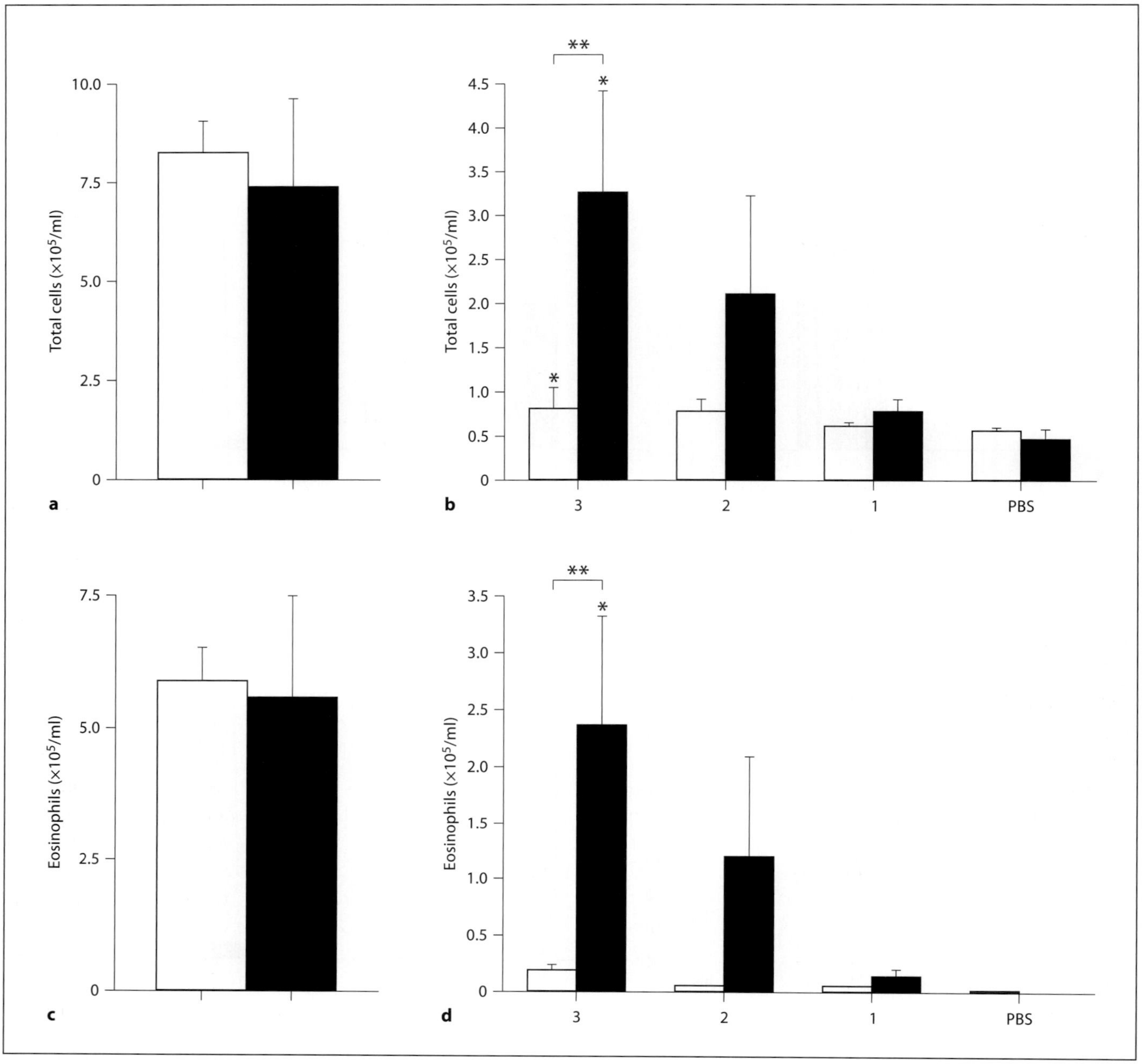

Fig. 2. Total cell (**a**, **b**) and eosinophil (**c**, **d**) counts in BALF. BALB/c mice (□) or C57BL/6 mice (■) were sensitized intraperitoneally to OVA with the adjuvant, alum (**a**, **c**), or epicutaneously (1–3 times) without adjuvant (**b**, **d**) for 3 weeks and then exposed to aerosolized OVA. Some mice were treated with skin patches containing PBS alone (PBS). Means ± SEM. n = 4–16. * $p < 0.005$ vs. animals sensitized epicutaneously with PBS, ** $p < 0.05$ between strains.

tized epicutaneously, increasing as a function of the number of allergen sensitizations ($n = 4–6$, $p < 0.005$). In epicutaneously sensitized animals, serum concentrations of IgG1 were significantly higher in BALB/c than in C57BL/6 mice ($p < 0.05$; fig. 1b). OVA-specific IgE was only detected in the serum of BALB/c mice sensitized systemically or epicutaneously (fig. 1c, d).

Exposure of sensitized animals to an inhaled allergen causes an eosinophil-dominant inflammation of the airways. As was observed with the production of allergen-

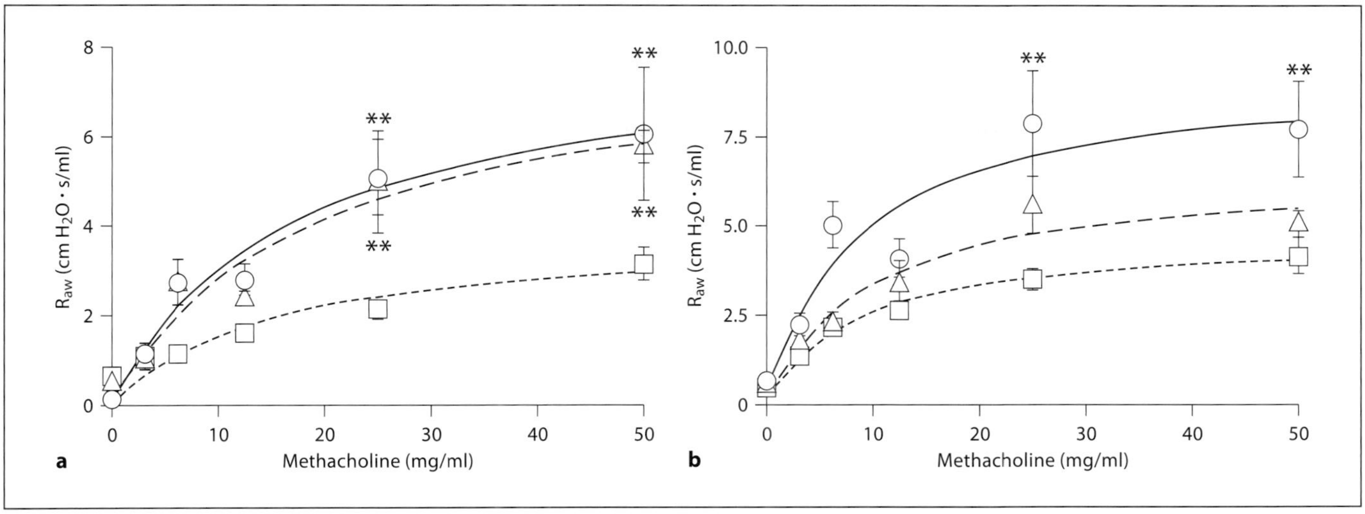

Fig. 3. Concentration-response curves of airway resistance (R_{aw}) to inhaled methacholine. C57BL/6 mice (**a**) or BALB/c mice (**b**) were sensitized to OVA intraperitoneally (——) or epicutaneously (– – –) or sensitized to PBS epicutaneously (------) for 3 weeks, then exposed to aerosolized OVA. Means ± SEM. n = 4–5. ** $p < 0.01$ vs. animals sensitized epicutaneously with PBS.

specific IgG1, the overall number of inflammatory cells and the number of eosinophils in BALF was similar in BALB/c and C57BL/6 mice sensitized intraperitoneally (fig. 2). In contrast, significant differences were found in the number of inflammatory cells and eosinophils in BALF between the two strains sensitized epicutaneously. It is noteworthy that, in contrast to the changes observed in allergen-specific IgG1 synthesis, the total cell and eosinophil counts were significantly higher in C57BL/6 than in BALB/c mice ($p < 0.05$, fig. 2).

We then examined airway responsiveness to methacholine in sedated, ventilated mice, 24 h after exposure to the last dose of inhaled OVA. Intraperitoneal sensitization following exposure of the airways to the allergen elicited hyperresponsiveness to methacholine in both BALB/c and C57BL/6 mice ($p < 0.01$; fig. 3). A similar degree of airway hyperresponsiveness to methacholine was observed in C57BL/6 mice sensitized epicutaneously ($p < 0.01$; fig. 3a); in contrast, BALB/c mice sensitized epicutaneously with OVA exhibited responses to methacholine similar to those observed in PBS-treated animals (fig. 3b).

To identify the immunological differences associated with specific phenotypes in BALB/c and C57BL/6 mice, we analyzed the cytokine composition of their BALF and compared it with that found in PBS-treated mice. The BALF concentrations of Th2 cytokines, including IL-4, IL-5 and IL-13, were increased in both the intraperitoneally sensitized BALB/c and in the similarly treated C57BL/6 mice (fig. 4a–c). In C57BL/6 mice sensitized epicutaneously, IL-4 levels in the BALF were significantly higher than in the samples obtained from PBS-treated, allergen-exposed animals (n = 4, $p < 0.001$, fig. 4a); there was a modest increase in IL-5 levels, but the concentration of IL-13 was unchanged (fig. 4b, c). In contrast, IL-4, IL-5 or IL-13 concentrations did not significantly change in the epicutaneously sensitized BALB/c mice. The difference in IL-4 levels between epicutaneously sensitized BALB/c mice and C57BL/6 mice was statistically significant (n = 4, $p < 0.001$, fig. 4a). IFN-γ (fig. 4d) or IL-12 (p70) and IL-17 (data not shown) concentrations did not differ between the PBS-treated mice and either strain of OVA-sensitized mice irrespective of the route of sensitization (intraperitoneally or epicutaneously).

Discussion

Following the intraperitoneal sensitization of BALB/c and C57BL/6 mice with OVA, (a) the antigen-specific IgG1 production, (b) the degree of eosinophilic airway inflammation, (c) bronchial responsiveness to methacholine and (d) cytokine production were similar in both strains. In contrast, after epicutaneous sensitization, eosinophilic inflammation of the airways and bronchial hy-

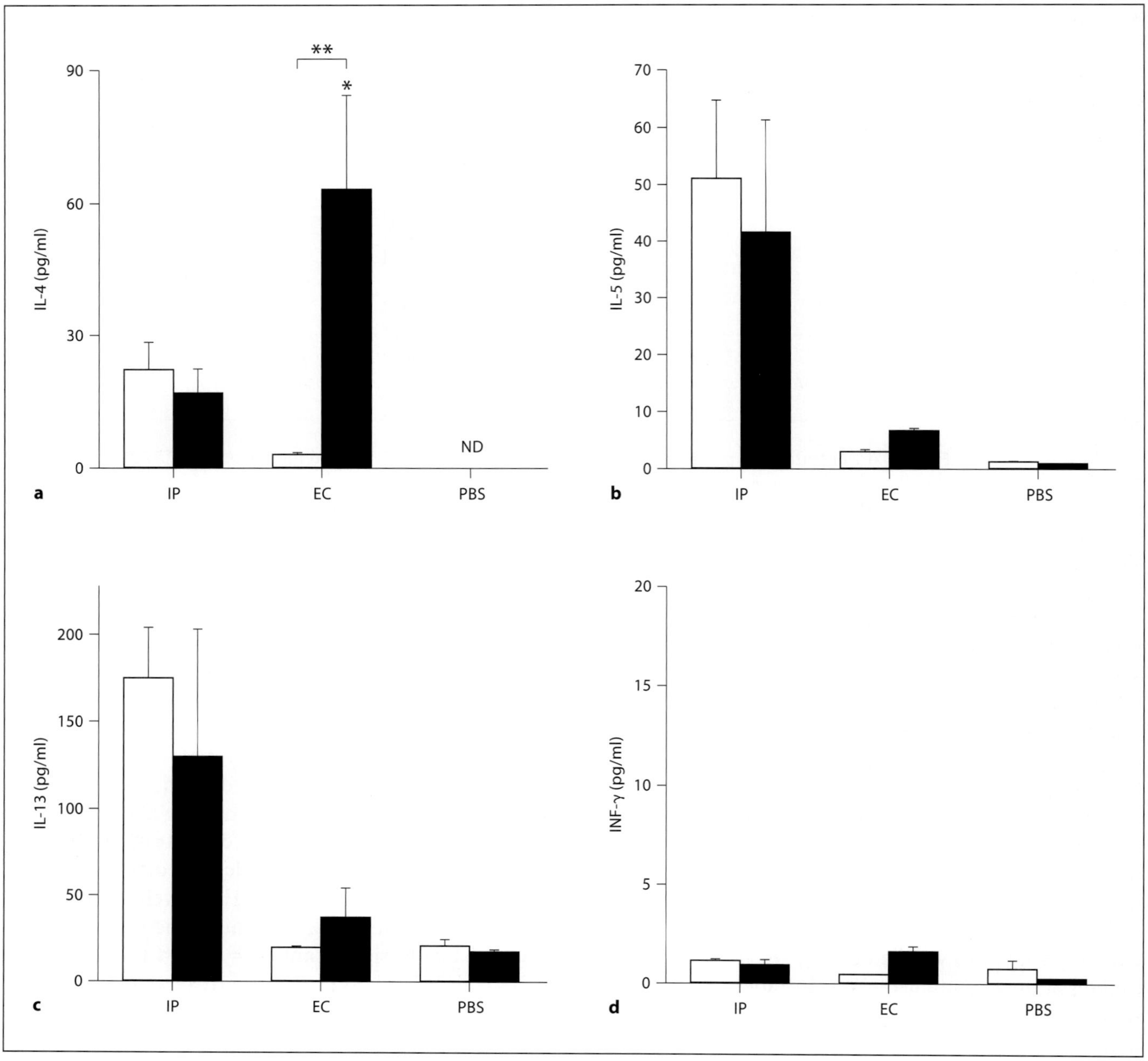

Fig. 4. Concentrations of IL-4 (**a**), IL-5 (**b**), IL-13 (**c**) and IFN-γ (**d**) in BALF. BALB/c mice (□) or C57BL/6 mice (■) were sensitized to OVA intraperitoneally (IP) or epicutaneously (EC) or sensitized to PBS epicutaneously (PBS) for 3 weeks and then exposed to aerosolized OVA. ND = Not detected. Means ± SEM. n = 4. * $p < 0.001$ vs. mice sensitized epicutaneously with PBS, ** $p < 0.001$ between strains.

perresponsiveness were significantly more prominent in C57BL/6 than in BALB/c mice, while the allergen-specific production of IgG1 and IgE was significantly greater in BALB/c than in C57BL/6 mice.

BALB/c and C57BL/6 mice are generally considered to be high and low producers of IgE [11, 12], respectively. This observation was confirmed by the higher concentrations of allergen-specific IgG1 and IgE found in the BALB/c mice sensitized epicutaneously compared with the C57BL/6 mice. After repeated exposure of the airways to the allergen, however, eosinophilic inflammation of the lungs and bronchial responsiveness to methacholine were more prominent in C57BL/6 than in BALB/c mice. Our analysis of the cytokine concentrations in the lungs explained this inconsistency. Specifically, we measured significantly higher concentrations of IL-4 in the BALF of epicutaneously sensitized C57BL/6 than in BALB/c mice. Morokata et al. [12] also reported higher IL-4 levels in BALF from allergen-exposed C57BL/6 mice than from BALB/c mice, while splenocytes from BALB/c mice stimulated with allergen in vitro had higher IL-4 levels than those from C57BL/6 mice. These findings suggest that local immune responses in the airways are critical determinants of the severity of airway inflammation and bronchial responsiveness, while the amount of Ig synthesized may be critically determined by systemic immune responses.

The bronchial responsiveness to methacholine was significantly greater in the epicutaneously sensitized C57BL/6 than in the PBS-sensitized mice. In contrast, we observed no significant increase in the bronchial responsiveness of BALB/c mice sensitized epicutaneously, while intraperitoneal sensitization followed by challenge with an aerosolized allergen induced a similarly prominent bronchial hyperresponsiveness in both mice strains. These observations suggest that C57BL/6 mice are more reliable to study the bronchial response to epicutaneous sensitization. In previous studies, the cutaneous challenge followed by inhalation of aerosolized OVA induced bronchial hyperresponsiveness in BALB/c mice [7, 8, 13, 14]. However, in most studies [7, 13, 14], enhanced pause (Penh), a dimensionless quantity that does not distinguish upper from lower airway responses, and whose physiological significance in mice has been questioned [15–17], was used to measure bronchial responsiveness. Another study [8], which used standard body plethysmography to measure bronchial responsiveness, found a minimal difference between OVA-exposed and control mice.

In our epicutaneous sensitization model, Th2-type responses occurred in the absence of concomitant adjuvant, such as alum, while it was indispensable in the intraperitoneal sensitization protocol, suggesting that the skin is a strong immunogenic organ that shows a Th2-deviated response to exogenous allergen. Indeed, acute removal of the skin barrier alone was capable of inducing the expression of Th2 chemokines, such as CCL17/TARC and CCL22/MDC, by epidermal cells [18]. Another possible explanation for the adjuvant-free sensitization observed in our model might be a minute contamination by pathogen-associated molecules, including fungi, mycoplasma-associated lipopeptide, histamine or prostaglandins, that function as Th2 adjuvants. Further studies are needed to clarify by which mechanisms the immunological responses are skewed toward Th2 dominance following epicutaneous sensitization.

In conclusion, we have created a reliable asthma model that uses a skin-mediated sensitization protocol, associated with increased allergen-specific immunoglobulin synthesis, eosinophilic airway inflammation and bronchial hyperresponsiveness, and found that C57BL/6 mice most appropriately fit this model. This will help clarify the relationship between skin barrier dysfunction and the pathogenesis of allergic asthma.

Acknowledgments

This study was supported by grants-in-aid for scientific research from the Ministries of Education, Science and Culture, and of Health, Labor and Welfare of Japan.

Disclosure Statement

The authors declare that no financial or other conflict of interest exists in relation to the content of this article.

References

1 Leung DY: Preface to atopic dermatitis intervention to control the atopic march. J Allergy Clin Immunol 2003;112(6 suppl):S117.

2 Spergel JM, Paller AS: Atopic dermatitis and the atopic march. J Allergy Clin Immunol 2003;112:(6 suppl)S118–S127.

3 Palmer CN, Irvine AD, Terron-Kwiatkowski A, Zhao Y, Liao H, Lee SP, Goudie DR, Sandilands A, Campbell LE, Smith FJ, O'Regan GM, Watson RM, Cecil JE, Bale SJ, Compton JG, DiGiovanna JJ, Fleckman P, Lewis-Jones S, Arseculeratne G, Sergeant A, Munro CS, El Houate B, McElreavey K, Halkjaer LB, Bisgaard H, Mukhopadhyay S, McLean WH: Common loss-of-function variants of the epidermal barrier protein filaggrin are a major predisposing factor for atopic dermatitis. Nat Genet 2006;38:441–446.

4 Weidinger S, Illig T, Baurecht H, Irvine AD, Rodriguez E, Diaz-Lacava A, Klopp N, Wagenpfeil S, Zhao Y, Liao H, Lee SP, Palmer CN, Jenneck C, Maintz L, Hagemann T, Behrendt H, Ring J, Nothen MM, McLean WH, Novak N: Loss-of-function variations within the filaggrin gene predispose for atopic dermatitis with allergic sensitizations. J Allergy Clin Immunol 2006;118:214–219.

5 Palmer CN, Ismail T, Lee SP, Terron-Kwiatkowski A, Zhao Y, Liao H, Smith FJ, McLean WH, Mukhopadhyay S: Filaggrin null mutations are associated with increased asthma severity in children and young adults. J Allergy Clin Immunol 2007;120:64–68.
6 Berard F, Marty JP, Nicolas JF: Allergen penetration through the skin. Eur J Dermatol 2003;13:324–330.
7 Akei HS, Brandt EB, Mishra A, Strait RT, Finkelman FD, Warrier MR, Hershey GK, Blanchard C, Rothenberg ME: Epicutaneous aeroallergen exposure induces systemic TH2 immunity that predisposes to allergic nasal responses. J Allergy Clin Immunol 2006;118: 62–69.
8 Spergel JM, Mizoguchi E, Brewer JP, Martin TR, Bhan AK, Geha RS: Epicutaneous sensitization with protein antigen induces localized allergic dermatitis and hyperresponsiveness to methacholine after single exposure to aerosolized antigen in mice. J Clin Invest 1998;101:1614–1622.
9 Wang LF, Lin JY, Hsieh KH, Lin RH: Epicutaneous exposure of protein antigen induces a predominant Th2-like response with high IgE production in mice. J Immunol 1996; 156:4077–4082.
10 Akei HS, Mishra A, Blanchard C, Rothenberg ME: Epicutaneous antigen exposure primes for experimental eosinophilic esophagitis in mice. Gastroenterology 2005;129: 985–994.
11 Herz U, Braun A, Rückert R, Renz H: Various immunological phenotypes are associated with increased airway responsiveness. Clin Exp Allergy 1998;28:625–634.
12 Morokata T, Ishikawa J, Ida K, Yamada T: C57BL/6 mice are more susceptible to antigen-induced pulmonary eosinophilia than BALB/c mice, irrespective of systemic T helper 1/T helper 2 responses. Immunology 1999;98:345–351.
13 He R, Oyoshi MK, Jin H, Geha RS: Epicutaneous antigen exposure induces a Th17 response that drives airway inflammation after inhalation challenge. Proc Natl Acad Sci USA 2007;104:15817–15822.
14 Ma W, Bryce PJ, Humbles AA, Laouini D, Yalcindag A, Alenius H, Friend DS, Oettgen HC, Gerard C, Geha RS: CCR3 is essential for skin eosinophilia and airway hyperresponsiveness in a murine model of allergic skin inflammation. J Clin Invest 2002;109: 621–628.
15 Adler A, Cieslewicz G, Irvin CG: Unrestrained plethysmography is an unreliable measure of airway responsiveness in BALB/c and C57BL/6 mice. J Appl Physiol 2004;97: 286–292.
16 Petak F, Habre W, Donati YR, Hantos Z, Barazzone-Argiroffo C: Hyperoxia-induced changes in mouse lung mechanics: forced oscillations vs. barometric plethysmography. J Appl Physiol 2001;90:2221–2230.
17 Bates J, Irvin C, Brusasco V, Drazen J, Fredberg J, Loring S, Eidelman D, Ludwig M, Macklem P, Martin J, Milic-Emili J, Hantos Z, Hyatt R, Lai-Fook S, Leff A, Solway J, Lutchen K, Suki B, Mitzner W, Paré P, Pride N, Sly P: The use and misuse of Penh in animal models of lung disease. Am J Respir Cell Mol Biol 2004;31:373–374.
18 Onoue A, Kabashima K, Kobayashi M, Mori T, Tokura Y: Induction of eosinophil- and Th2-attracting epidermal chemokines and cutaneous late-phase reaction in tape-stripped skin. Exp Dermatol 2009;18:1036–1043.

Original Paper

International Archives of Allergy and Immunology

Int Arch Allergy Immunol 2010;152(suppl 1):75–78
DOI: 10.1159/000312129

Published online: June 4, 2010

Effect of Sublingual Immunotherapy on Antigen-Induced Bronchial and Nasal Inflammation in Mice

Osamu Kaminuma[a, b] Kazuya Suzuki[b] Akio Mori[a]

[a]Clinical Research Center for Allergy and Rheumatology, National Hospital Organization, Sagamihara National Hospital, Kanagawa, and [b]Department of Allergy and Immunology, Tokyo Metropolitan Institute of Medical Science, Tokyo, Japan

Key Words

Airway inflammation · Asthma · Neutrophils · Rhinitis · Sublingual immunotherapy

Abstract

Background: Sublingual immunotherapy (SLIT) is effective in the treatment of a variety of allergic diseases, including bronchial asthma and rhinitis. However, how this local therapy exerts such wide effects is unclear. In this study, we comparatively examined the effect of SLIT on antigen-induced airway inflammation in bronchoalveolar and nasal cavities in mice. ***Methods:*** Mice were treated sublingually with ovalbumin (OVA) once a day for 2 weeks. Subsequently, they were immunized with the corresponding antigen. Following intratracheal and nasal challenge with OVA, infiltration of inflammatory cells into the bronchoalveolar and nasal cavities was investigated in these mice. ***Results:*** Massive infiltration of eosinophils as well as neutrophils into the bronchoalveolar cavity was induced by intratracheal OVA challenge. Eosinophils accumulated in the nasal cavity, but the number of neutrophils did not significantly change in response to nasal antigen challenge. These antigen-induced airway inflammatory responses, including the increases in the numbers of eosinophils and/or neutrophils in the bronchoalveolar and nasal cavities, were clearly suppressed by SLIT. ***Conclusions:*** This animal model displaying differential inflammatory responses in the bronchoalveolar and nasal cavities may be useful to elucidate the efficacy and mechanisms of SLIT against various allergic diseases.

Introduction

Accumulating evidence suggests that antigen-specific immunotherapy is an effective means to treat allergic disorders. To carry out this therapy, patients are sensitized to a small amount of antigens administered mainly via the subcutaneous route [1]. In order to relieve the discomfort of patients receiving long-term and frequent antigen injections, some alternative administration routes, such as oral and nasal administration, have been examined recently. Especially, sublingual immunotherapy (SLIT) is one of the most promising treatments because of its high efficiency and non-invasiveness [2, 3]. Since the distribution of antigen administered is limited, the frequency of adverse effects elicited by SLIT is very low [4]. Nonetheless, this local therapy shows strong efficacy against allergic diseases developed in a variety of target organs [4].

KARGER

Fax +41 61 306 12 34
E-Mail karger@karger.ch
www.karger.com

1018–2438/10/1525–0075$26.00/0

Accessible online at:
www.karger.com/iaa

Correspondence to: Dr. Akio Mori
National Hospital Organization, Sagamihara National Hospital
Clinical Research Center for Allergy and Rheumatology
18-1 Sakuradai, Sagamihara, Kanagawa 228-8522 (Japan)
Tel. +81 42 742 8311, Fax +81 42 742 7990, E-Mail mori-kkr@umin.ac.jp

Along with the alleviation of local allergic symptoms, SLIT causes several systemic responses. For example, the level of serum antigen-specific IgG4, which reflects Th1 response, was increased following the treatment of SLIT [5]. However, how this immunotherapy shows strong efficacy against various allergic diseases has not been fully elucidated yet.

So far, few animal models mimicking SLIT for the treatment of allergic diseases have been reported [6, 7]. Sublingual administration of a specific antigen to immunized mice prevented antigen-induced IgE production, infiltration of eosinophils into the nasal cavity, sneezing and bronchial hyperreactivity [6]. In addition, antigen-specific IgA was drastically increased, whereas IgE was undetectable in the bronchoalveolar lavage (BAL) fluid (BALF) and nasal lavage (NAL) fluid (NALF) after repeated sublingual antigen administration [7]. Even though these animal models are useful to elucidate the efficacy and mechanisms of SLIT, it has not been clarified whether SLIT differentially modulates antigen-specific responses among target organs or not. In this report, we comparatively investigated the effect of SLIT against antigen-induced airway inflammation in both the bronchoalveolar and nasal cavities in mice.

Methods

Sublingual Administration and Immunization with Ovalbumin

Female 6- to 8-week-old BALB/c mice were lightly anesthetized with diethyl ether and sublingually administered ovalbumin (OVA) or PBS (control) by holding the scruff, carefully applying 10 μl of OVA solution (100 mg/ml) under the tongue daily for 14 days. Then, mice were immunized with two intraperitoneal injections of alum-absorbed OVA (20 μg) on days 15 and 29.

Antigen Challenge and Assessment of Airway Inflammation

Mice were lightly anesthetized with pentobarbital (Dainippon, Osaka, Japan) and intratracheally challenged with 10 μg of OVA on day 43, and BAL was performed on day 45. For NAL analysis, mice were intranasally challenged once a day with 20 μg of OVA from days 43 to 47 consecutively, and NAL was performed on day 48. The numbers of inflammatory cells recovered in the BALF and NALF were counted by hemocytometer and differential cell counts prepared by cytospins were performed as described previously [8].

Statistical Analysis

Results are expressed as arithmetic means ± SEM. Statistical analysis was performed by one-way analysis of variance and Dunnet's method. $p < 0.05$ was considered to indicate statistical significance.

Results and Discussion

Prior to the evaluation of the effect of SLIT, immune responses of mice elicited by antigen immunization were examined. As shown in previous reports [6, 7], OVA-specific IgE and IgG were detectable in the serum of immunized mice. In addition, antigen-induced proliferation of splenic CD4+ T cells and production of Th2 cytokines, such as IL-4 and IL-5, by these cells were detectable after immunization with OVA (data not shown).

Next, the effect of SLIT on allergic inflammation induced in the bronchoalveolar and nasal cavities was investigated. Mice received OVA sublingually for 2 weeks and were immunized with the corresponding antigen. Then they were intratracheally or intranasally challenged with OVA. Large numbers of inflammatory cells, especially eosinophils and neutrophils, were recovered from the BALF of OVA-immunized and intratracheally challenged mice (fig. 1a). The antigen-induced increase in eosinophils was also observed in the NALF (fig. 1b), even though it was significant only after repeated OVA challenge. These responses were completely dependent on the specific antigen used for immunization and challenge. Thus, OVA challenge of mice immunized with a non-specific antigen, BSA, or BSA challenge of OVA-immunized mice did not induce the increase in inflammatory cells in the BALF as well as NALF (data not shown). A small number of neutrophils were observed in the nasal cavity of mice receiving PBS as a control, whereas this cell type was not significantly affected by immunization and provocation with the specific antigen (fig. 1b).

The infiltration of eosinophils and neutrophils into the bronchoalveolar cavity was significantly inhibited by sublingual administration of OVA. Eosinophil infiltration into the nasal cavity was also inhibited, but neutrophils were not affected by SLIT (fig. 1).

These findings are supported by previous investigations that production of antigen-specific immunoglobulins and CD4+ T-cell responses including Th2 proliferation and cytokine synthesis were suppressed by SLIT [6, 7]. The suppression of these responses was also observed in our experimental system (data not shown). Among Th2 cytokines, IL-5 plays a pivotal role in the development of eosinophilia [9, 10], i.e. the attenuation of antigen-induced accumulation of eosinophils both in the bronchoalveolar and nasal cavities by SLIT were possibly due, at least in part, to the down-regulation of IL-5 synthesis by CD4+ T cells.

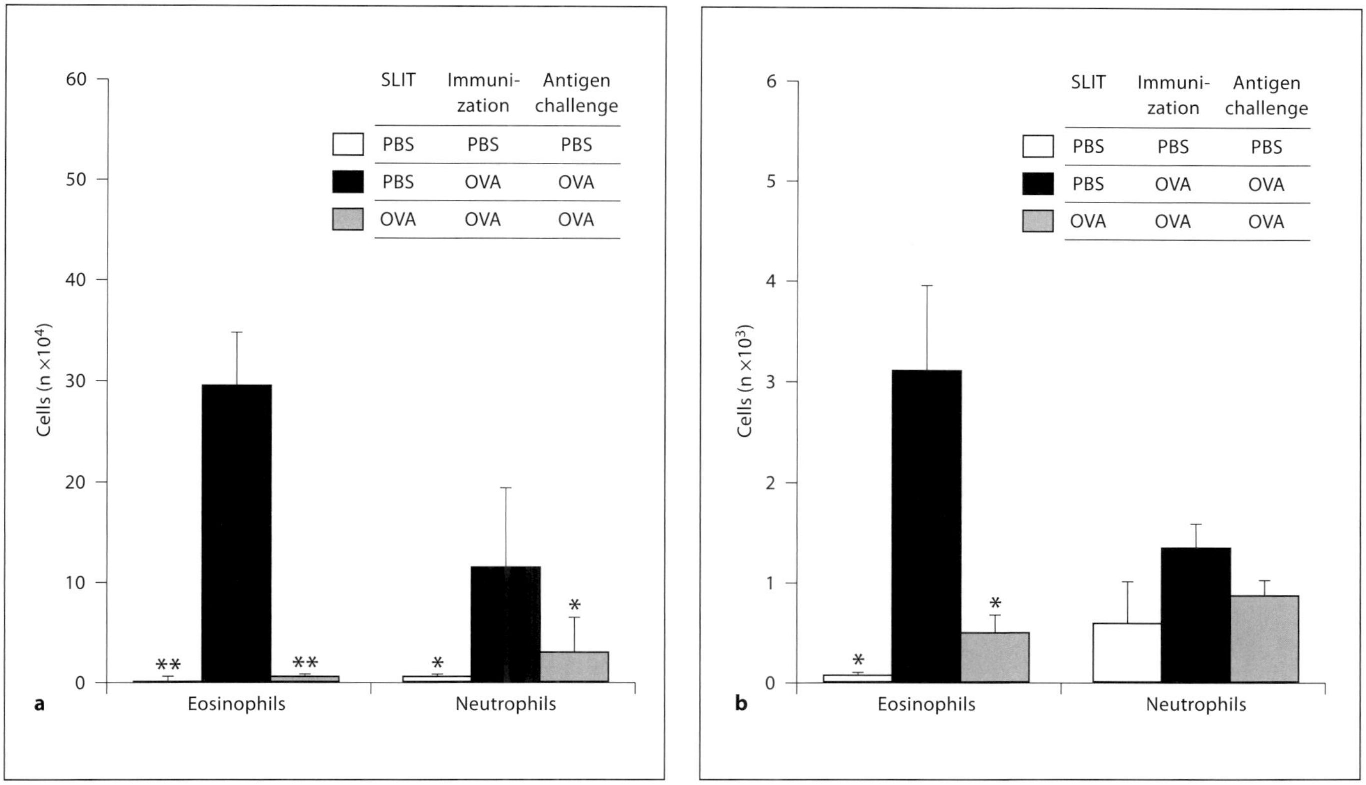

Fig. 1. Effect of SLIT on the infiltration of inflammatory cells into bronchoalveolar and nasal cavities. Mice received OVA sublingually once a day for 2 weeks. Then they were immunized with the corresponding antigen. After intratracheal and nasal challenge of mice with OVA, the numbers of eosinophils as well as neutrophils recovered in the BALF (**a**) and NALF (**b**), respectively, were determined. Means ± SEM of 5–6 animals for each group; * $p < 0.05$ and ** $p < 0.01$ vs. PBS group (control).

It is interesting that an increase in neutrophils was observed only in the bronchoalveolar cavity, even though antigen challenge procedures in BAL and NAL analyses were slightly different. Infiltration of neutrophils is regulated by several chemokines and chemotactic factors, such as CXCL1, CXCL2, CXCL8, platelet-activating factor and leukotriene B_4 [11–13]. Recently, Th17-mediated neutrophilic inflammation has also been implicated in allergic diseases [14]. Therefore, these neutrophil-reactive cytokines and/or other factors may be synthesized in response to antigen exposure in the bronchoalveolar but not nasal cavity. In order to elucidate additional details of the mechanisms underlying the difference between the bronchoalveolar and nasal cavity, a comparative analysis of neutrophil-activating factors produced in both organs is required and currently under investigation.

In conclusion, pathophysiological features of allergic inflammation developed in the bronchoalveolar and nasal cavity may be different. Our experimental system is potentially helpful to elucidate the mechanisms as well as effectiveness of SLIT in the treatment of a variety of allergic diseases.

Acknowledgments

The authors gratefully thank Dr. Takachika Hiroi for helpful discussions and suggestions. This work was supported in part by the Nisshin Seifun Foundation.

Disclosure Statement

The authors declare that no financial or other conflict of interest exists in relation to the content of this article.

References

1 Bousquet J, Lockey R, Malling HJ: Allergen immunotherapy: therapeutic vaccines for allergic diseases. A WHO position paper. J Allergy Clin Immunol 1998;102:558–562.

2 Potter PC: Update on sublingual immunotherapy. Ann Allergy Asthma Immunol 2006;96:S22–S25.

3 Cox LS, Larenas Linnemann D, Nolte H, Weldon D, Finegold I, Nelson HS: Sublingual immunotherapy: a comprehensive review. J Allergy Clin Immunol 2006;117:1021–1035.

4 Cox L: Allergen immunotherapy and asthma: efficacy, safety, and other considerations. Allergy Asthma Proc 2008;29:580–589.

5 Bousquet J, Scheinmann P, Guinnepain MT, Perrin-Fayolle M, Sauvaget J, Tonnel AB, Pauli G, Caillaud D, Dubost R, Leynadier F, Vervloet D, Herman D, Galvain S, Andre C: Sublingual-swallow immunotherapy (SLIT) in patients with asthma due to house-dust mites: a double-blind, placebo-controlled study. Allergy 1999;54:249–260.

6 Brimnes J, Kildsgaard J, Jacobi H, Lund K: Sublingual immunotherapy reduces allergic symptoms in a mouse model of rhinitis. Clin Exp Allergy 2007;37:488–497.

7 Kildsgaard J, Brimnes J, Jacobi H, Lund K: Sublingual immunotherapy in sensitized mice. Ann Allergy Asthma Immunol 2007; 98:366–372.

8 Suzuki K, Kaminuma O, Yang L, Motoi Y, Takai T, Ichikawa S, Okumura K, Ogawa H, Mori A, Takaiwa F, Hiroi T: Development of transgenic rice expressing mite antigen for a new concept of immunotherapy. Int Arch Allergy Immunol 2009;149(suppl 1):21–24.

9 Foster PS, Hogan SP, Ramsay AJ, Matthaei KI, Young IG: Interleukin 5 deficiency abolishes eosinophilia, airways hyperreactivity, and lung damage in a mouse asthma model. J Exp Med 1996;183:195–201.

10 Mauser PJ, Pitman A, Witt A, Fernandez X, Zurcher J, Kung T, Jones H, Watnick AS, Egan RW, Kreutner W, et al: Inhibitory effect of the TRFK-5 anti-IL-5 antibody in a guinea pig model of asthma. Am Rev Respir Dis 1993;148:1623–1627.

11 Gomez FP, Rodriguez-Roisin R: Platelet-activating factor antagonists: current status in asthma. BioDrugs 2000;14:21–30.

12 Ford-Hutchinson AW: Leukotriene B4 in inflammation. Crit Rev Immunol 1990;10:1–12.

13 Kobayashi Y: The role of chemokines in neutrophil biology. Front Biosci 2008;13:2400–2407.

14 Liang SC, Long AJ, Bennett F, Whitters MJ, Karim R, Collins M, Goldman SJ, Dunussi-Joannopoulos K, Williams CM, Wright JF, Fouser LA: An IL-17 F/A heterodimer protein is produced by mouse Th17 cells and induces airway neutrophil recruitment. J Immunol 2007;179:7791–7799.

Original Paper

International Archives of Allergy and Immunology

Int Arch Allergy Immunol 2010;152(suppl 1):79–82
DOI: 10.1159/000312130

Published online: June 4, 2010

Eosinophils Are Required for the Induction of Bronchial Hyperresponsiveness in a Th Transfer Model of BALB/c Background

Takayuki Ohtomo[a, b] Osamu Kaminuma[c] Junji Yamada[b] Noriko Kitamura[a] Akemi Abe[a] Noriaki Kobayashi[d] Matsunobu Suko[e] Akio Mori[a]

[a]National Hospital Organization, Sagamihara National Hospital, Clinical Research Center for Allergy and Rheumatology, Kanagawa, [b]Department of Pharmacotherapeutics, Tokyo University of Pharmacy and Life Sciences, [c]Tokyo Metropolitan Institute of Medical Science, and [d]Department of Biotechnology, Tokyo Technical College, and [e]Tokyo National University of Fine Arts and Music, Health Service Center, Tokyo, Japan

Key Words
Bronchial asthma · Bronchial hyperresponsiveness · Double GATA · Eosinophilic inflammation · Helper T cell

Abstract
Background: Helper T (Th) cells are deeply involved in the pathophysiology of bronchial asthma, such as eosinophilic inflammation, bronchial hyperresponsiveness (BHR), airflow limitation and remodeling. It is still unclear whether Th cells contribute to BHR independently of eosinophilic inflammation. The double GATA (dblGATA) site is a high-affinity GATA-binding site in the GATA-1 promoter. dblGATA site-deficient (ΔdblGATA) mice lack eosinophils. ***Method:*** Ovalbumin (OVA)-reactive Th clones were transferred into ΔdblGATA and wild-type (WT) mice of BALB/c background. The number of eosinophils in the bronchoalveolar lavage fluid (BALF) and bronchial responsiveness to methacholine were examined after OVA challenge. ***Results:*** The number of BALF eosinophils was significantly increased in WT mice, but not detectable in ΔdblGATA mice. BHR was also induced in WT mice, but significantly attenuated in ΔdblGATA mice. ***Conclusion:*** Eosinophils are involved in T-cell-mediated BHR.

Introduction

Eosinophilic inflammation and bronchial hyperresponsiveness (BHR) are the hallmarks of bronchial asthma, along with mucosal injury, excessive mucus production and airway remodeling. Airway eosinophilia was suppressed by the administration of anti-interleukin (IL)-5-neutralizing antibody, and abolished in IL-5-deficient mice, suggesting that IL-5 is indispensable for the development of eosinophilia [1–3]. IL-13 is essential for the development of BHR, as induction of BHR in murine asthma is totally inhibited by the administration of soluble IL-13 receptor-IgGFc fusion protein, which specifically binds to and neutralizes IL-13 [4, 5]. In addition, we and others studied adoptive transfer of helper T (Th)-cell-conferred eosinophilia and BHR to unprimed mice [6, 7], and results collectively indicate that both eosinophilia and BHR are mediated by Th cells.

The double GATA (dblGATA) site, which is a high-affinity GATA-binding site in the GATA-1 promoter, is located 500 bp upstream of the heterogeneous start sites of the GATA-1 gene [8]. Deletion of the dblGATA site leads to selective loss of the eosinophil lineage in vivo [9]. DblGATA-deficient (ΔdblGATA) mice of the BALB/c background were first established [10]. Eosinophil defi-

KARGER
Fax +41 61 306 12 34
E-Mail karger@karger.ch
www.karger.com

1018–2438/10/1525–0079$26.00/0

Accessible online at:
www.karger.com/iaa

Correspondence to: Dr. Akio Mori
National Hospital Organization, Sagamihara National Hospital
Clinical Research Center for Allergy and Rheumatology
18-1 Sakuradai, Sagamihara, Kanagawa 228-8522 (Japan)
Tel. +81 42 742 8311, Fax +81 42 742 7990, E-Mail mori-kkr@umin.ac.jp

ciency conferred no protection against BHR in ΔdblGATA mice immunized and challenged with allergen, suggesting that eosinophils are not obligatory for BHR. Later, ΔdblGATA mice of the C57BL/6 background were reported [11]. In quite contrast, after immunization and repeated antigen exposure, recruitment of $CD4^+$ cells to the lung was strongly attenuated compared to wild-type (WT) mice, and BHR was not induced. The discrepancy might be explained by the strain difference [11]. Moreover, induction of inflammation and BHR is affected not only by the genetic background of the experimental animals, but also by the models or experimental protocols used [12, 13]. Thus, it is not fully determined yet whether eosinophils are responsible for the development of BHR or not. We now examined the influence of eosinophil knockout in the induction of BHR employing an adoptive transfer model.

Materials and Methods

Animals

ΔdblGATA mice of BALB/c background and WT mice were used for the experiments. Mice were housed under specific pathogen-free conditions in an environmentally controlled clean room. All animal experiments were performed under protocols approved by the Animal Care and Use Committee of the Institute.

Establishment of Ovalbumin-Reactive T-Cell Clones

Establishment and maintenance of Th clones were performed as described previously [6]. Briefly, splenic T cells (2×10^6) were prepared from DO11.10 transgenic mice by passage through a nylon fiber column according to the method of Julius et al. [14], and cultured for 6–8 days in the presence of irradiated syngeneic spleen cells as antigen-presenting cells (6×10^6) and ovalbumin (OVA, 100 μg/ml). Cloning by limiting dilution was performed with the remaining viable cells in the presence of irradiated antigen-presenting cells, OVA and interleukin (IL)-2. After 2–3 weeks, positive wells were transferred to macrowells along with irradiated antigen-presenting cells, OVA and IL-2.

Cell Transfer and Challenge Procedures

Th clones (1×10^7) suspended in 0.3 ml of Hanks' balanced salt solution were injected into the tail vein of unprimed mice. Twenty-four hours later, mice were challenged intranasally with OVA (100 μg in 50 μl PBS). As a control, Th-clone-transferred mice were challenged with bovine serum albumin (BSA), and non-transferred mice were challenged with OVA.

Bronchoalveolar Lavage Procedures

Bronchoalveolar lavage (BAL) was performed as reported previously [15]. Briefly, the trachea was cannulated with a polyethylene tube through which the lungs were gently lavaged with 0.4 ml of HBSS 5 times (2 ml total). On average, 1.9 ml BAL fluid (BALF) was recovered and then centrifuged. Differential cell counts were made by microscopic examination of centrifuged preparations stained with May-Giemsa, counting 200 cells in each animal.

Measurement of BHR

For measurement of intubated lung resistance (R_L), mice were anesthetized with intraperitoneal injection of pentobarbital (50 mg/kg), vecuronium bromide (0.2 mg/kg) and xylazine (2 mg/kg) to block spontaneous breathing under anesthesia. Mice were mechanically ventilated at 170 breaths/min with a tidal volume of 6 ml/kg. One port of a 4-way connector was attached to the tracheotomy tube, and the other two ports were attached to the inspiratory and expiratory side of the ventilator. Aerosolized methacholine was administered for 10 s with a tidal volume of 10 μl, with airflow calculated from the pressure changes in the plethysmograph by BioSystem XA software. Mean R_L was calculated from a 3-min measurement after administration of inhaled methacholine at 1.6–6.3 mg/ml.

Statistical Analysis

Results are presented as means ± SEM. Statistical analysis was performed with ANOVA. To test differences between individual groups, Student's t test was performed and $p < 0.05$ was considered statistically significant.

Results and Discussion

To examine the effect of dblGATA deficiency on eosinophil recruitment following antigen challenge in our adoptive Th transfer asthma model, OVA-reactive Th clones (BF7) were transferred into unprimed ΔdblGATA and WT mice of BALB/c background, and mice were challenged with antigen. BALF eosinophilia 48 h after OVA challenge was first compared (fig. 1). The numbers of eosinophils, neutrophils, lymphocytes and monocytes/macrophages in the BALF of BF7-transferred WT mice were increased upon antigen challenge approximately 8.0-, 4.0-, 16.8- and 3.0-fold, respectively. The numbers of neutrophils, lymphocytes and monocytes/macrophages in the BALF of BF7-transferred ΔdblGATA mice were increased upon antigen challenge 10.3-, 17.6- and 3.1-fold, respectively, and eosinophils were not detectable. Infiltration of neutrophils, lymphocytes and monocytes/macrophages was induced in quite equivalent magnitude between WT and ΔdblGATA mice, indicating that the ΔdblGATA mutation was selective for eosinophils. Our present experiment clearly demonstrated that disruption of the dblGATA site ameliorated eosinophilia in Th-transferred mice, consistent with the previous reports that employed actively sensitized BALB/c mice [10, 11].

The role of eosinophils in the development of BHR was next examined. R_L of BF7-transferred ΔdblGATA and WT mice was measured using a Buxco BioSystem plethysmograph. BHR was quantified in response to increasing doses of methacholine. As shown in figure 2, R_L values of BF7-transferred WT mice challenged with OVA

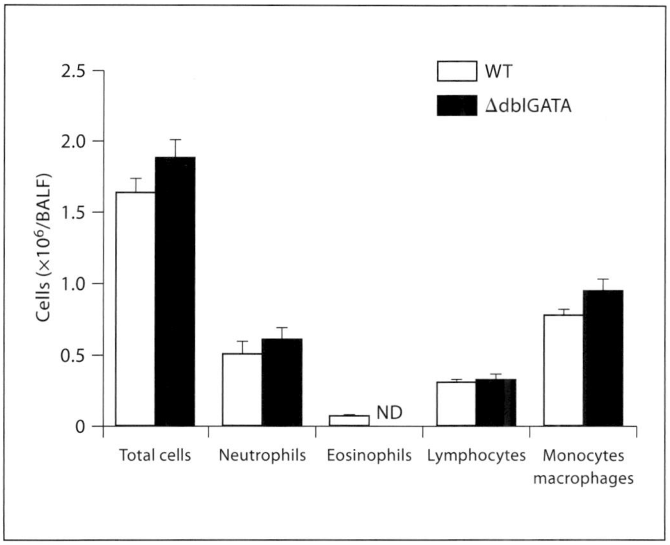

Fig. 1. Numbers of infiltrating cells in BALF of Th-transferred BALB/c mice challenged with OVA. The numbers of total cells, neutrophils, eosinophils, lymphocytes and monocytes/macrophages (Mø) of WT mice were 1.62×10^6, 4.94×10^5, 6.09×10^4, 3.00×10^5 and 7.67×10^5, respectively. The numbers of total cells, neutrophils, lymphocytes and monocytes/macrophages of ΔdblGATA mice were 1.88×10^6, 6.01×10^5, 3.20×10^5 and 9.39×10^5, respectively. Eosinophils of ΔdblGATA mice were not detectable. Means ± SEM. Each experimental group consisted of >3 animals. ND = Not detectable.

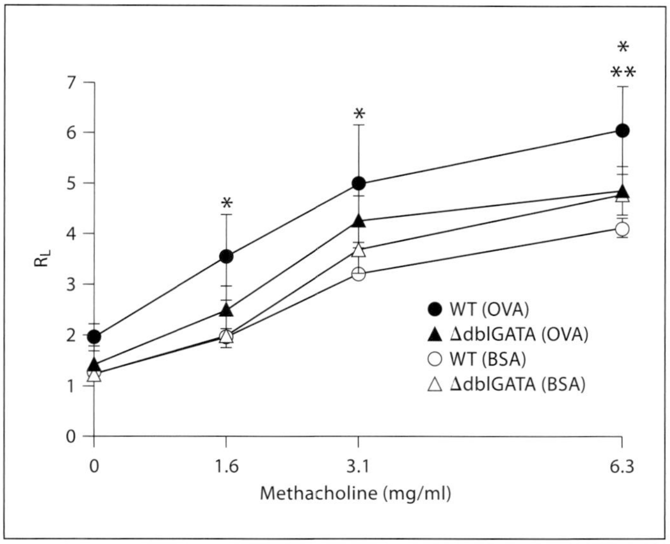

Fig. 2. Eosinophils are required for the development of BHR in response to antigen in Th-transferred BALB/c mice. An OVA-reactive Th clone, BF7, was established from splenic T cells of DO11.10 mice. Unprimed BALB/c WT and ΔdblGATA mice were transferred intravenously with BF7 (1×10^7 cells) and challenged with OVA. As a control, BF7-transferred WT and ΔdblGATA mice were challenged with BSA, respectively. R_L was recorded for individual animals 48 h after challenge. R_L values of BF7-transferred WT and ΔdblGATA mice challenged with OVA, and BF7-transferred WT and ΔdblGATA mice challenged with BSA were 6.13, 4.87, 4.85 and 4.18 after inhalation of 6.3 mg/ml methacholine, respectively. Means ± SEM. Each experimental group consisted of >3 animals. * $p < 0.05$, compared with WT mice challenged with BSA, ** $p < 0.05$, compared with ΔdblGATA mice challenged with OVA.

(●) corresponding to each methacholine concentration was significantly increased compared to those of BSA-challenged WT mice (○, * $p < 0.05$), consistent with our previous report [15]. R_L values of BF7-transferred dblGATA mice challenged with OVA (▲) were not significantly increased compared to those of BSA-challenged ΔdblGATA mice (△), and were significantly less than that of WT mice (●, ** $p < 0.05$). The finding clearly indicated that the induction of BHR was abolished by eosinophil deficiency.

Bronchial asthma is a chronic disorder characterized by persistent airway inflammation with marked eosinophilia and BHR. In regard to the relationship between eosinophilia and BHR, two contrasting reports on experimental asthma have been made so far [10, 11]. On the C57BL/6 background, eosinophils are mandatory for the induction of BHR, whereas BHR is induced in the absence of eosinophils on the BALB/c background [10, 11]. To reconcile the apparent discrepancy, strain-specific requirements of eosinophils were proposed for the development of BHR, i.e. different magnitudes of T-cell recruitment to the lung [11]. BALB/c represents a high Th2 responder compared with C57BL/6 in terms of higher IgE responses and airway responsiveness after allergen challenge [12, 13]. To investigate the role of Th cells more directly, a murine asthma model employing adoptive transfer of Th clones has been reported, and eosinophilia [6], BHR [16] and airway remodeling [17] were induced upon antigen challenge in Th2-transferred mice independently of humoral immune responses. Our present study employed a Th transfer model and clearly demonstrated that eosinophils are obligatory for the induction of BHR on the BALB/c background for the first time. Our finding is consistent with the report made by Walsh et al. [11] on the C57BL/6 background. With respect to the BALB/c background, Humbles et al. [10] reported that BHR was equally induced in ΔdblGATA and WT mice actively sensitized and challenged with antigen. The reason for the apparent discrepancy between the two studies is not fully clear at this moment, but IgE antibody might play some role in the induction of BHR through the activation of mast cells, a significant source of inflammatory mediators and cytokines including IL-4, TNF-α and leukotrienes, for example [18, 19], since BALB/c mice displayed greater mast cell infiltration into the lung compared to C57BL/6 mice after immunization and antigen exposure [20]. It is pretty intriguing to determine whether BHR would resume upon further supplementation of humoral immunity by the infusion of antigen-specific IgE, IgG or IgA antibodies in addition to Th cells.

In conclusion, our study clearly demonstrated that eosinophils play a critical role in Th-mediated BHR in mice of BALB/c background for the first time. Eosinophil-targeted therapy might be of considerable interest in controlling T-cell-mediated features of asthma.

Acknowledgments

This work was supported in part by Health and Labor Science Research Grants for Research on Allergic Disease and Immunology (A.M.), the Program for the Promotion of Fundamental Studies in Health Science of the National Institute of Biomedical Innovation (A.M.) and a grant from the Charitable Trust Clinical Pathology Research Foundation of Japan (A.M.).

Disclosure Statement

The authors declare that no financial or other conflict of interest exists in relation to the content of this article.

References

1 Mauser PJ, Pitman A, Witt A, Fernandez X, Zurcher J, Kung T, Jones H, Watnick AS, Egan RW, Kreutner W, et al: Inhibitory effect of the TRFK-5 anti-IL-5 antibody in a guinea pig model of asthma. Am Rev Respir Dis 1993;148:1623–1627.

2 Foster PS, Hogan SP, Ramsay AJ, Matthaei KI, Young IG: Interleukin 5 deficiency abolishes eosinophilia, airways hyperreactivity, and lung damage in a mouse asthma model. J Exp Med 1996;183:195–201.

3 Nakajima H, Iwamoto I, Tomoe S, Matsumura R, Tomioka H, Takatsu K, Yoshida S: CD4+ T-lymphocytes and interleukin-5 mediate antigen-induced eosinophil infiltration into the mouse trachea. Am Rev Respir Dis 1992;146:374–377.

4 Wills-Karp M, Luyimbazi J, Xu X, Schofield B, Neben TY, Karp CL, Donaldson DD: Interleukin-13: central mediator of allergic asthma. Science 1998;282:2258–2261.

5 Grunig G, Warnock M, Wakil AE, Venkayya R, Brombacher F, Rennick DM, Sheppard D, Mohrs M, Donaldson DD, Locksley RM, Corry DB: Requirement for IL-13 independently of IL-4 in experimental asthma. Science 1998;282:2261–2263.

6 Kaminuma O, Mori A, Ogawa K, Nakata A, Kikkawa H, Naito K, Suko M, Okudaira H: Successful transfer of late phase eosinophil infiltration in the lung by infusion of helper T cell clones. Am J Respir Cell Mol Biol 1997; 16:448–454.

7 Ohtomo T, Kaminuma O, Kitamura N, Suko M, Kobayashi N, Mori A: Murine Th clones confer late asthmatic response upon antigen challenge. Int Arch Allergy Immunol 2009; 149(suppl 1):2–6.

8 Tsai SF, Strauss E, Orkin SH: Functional analysis and in vivo footprinting implicate the erythroid transcription factor GATA-1 as a positive regulator of its own promoter. Genes Dev 1991;5:919–931.

9 Yu C, Cantor AB, Yang H, Browne C, Wells RA, Fujiwara Y, Orkin SH: Targeted deletion of a high-affinity GATA-binding site in the GATA-1 promoter leads to selective loss of the eosinophil lineage in vivo. J Exp Med 2002;195:1387–1395.

10 Humbles AA, Lloyd CM, McMillan SJ, Friend DS, Xanthou G, McKenna EE, Ghiran S, Gerard NP, Yu C, Orkin SH, Gerard C: A critical role for eosinophils in allergic airways remodeling. Science 2004;305:1776–1779.

11 Walsh ER, Sahu N, Kearley J, Benjamin E, Kang BH, Humbles A, August A: Strain-specific requirement for eosinophils in the recruitment of T cells to the lung during the development of allergic asthma. J Exp Med 2008;205:1285–1292.

12 Takeda K, Haczku A, Lee JJ, Irvin CG, Gelfand EW: Strain dependence of airway hyperresponsiveness reflects differences in eosinophil localization in the lung. Am J Physiol Lung Cell Mol Physiol 2001; 281:L394–L402.

13 Singh B, Shinagawa K, Taube C, Gelfand EW, Pabst R: Strain-specific differences in perivascular inflammation in lungs in two murine models of allergic airway inflammation. Clin Exp Immunol 2005;141:223–229.

14 Julius MH, Simpson E, Herzenberg LA: A rapid method for the isolation of functional thymus-derived murine lymphocytes. Eur J Immunol 1973;3:645–649.

15 Ohtomo T, Miyatake S, Kajiyama Y, Umezu-Goto M, Kobayashi N, Kaminuma O, Mori A: Airway eosinophilic inflammation is attenuated in conserved noncoding sequence-1-deficient mice. Int Arch Allergy Immunol 2008;146(suppl 1):2–6.

16 Nakata A, Kaminuma O, Ogawa K, Fujimura H, Fushimi K, Kikkawa H, Naito K, Ikezawa K, Egan RW, Mori A: Correlation between eosinophilia induced by CD4(+) T cells and bronchial hyper-responsiveness. Int Immunol 2001;13:329–339.

17 Kaminuma O, Fujimura H, Fushimi K, Nakata A, Sakai A, Chishima S, Ogawa K, Kikuchi M, Kikkawa H, Akiyama K, Mori A: Dynamics of antigen-specific helper T cells at the initiation of airway eosinophilic inflammation. Eur J Immunol 2001;31:2669–2679.

18 Jeffery PK, Haahtela T: Allergic rhinitis and asthma: inflammation in a one-airway condition (review). BMC Pulm Med 2006;6(suppl 1):S5.

19 Brightling CE, Symon FA, Holgate ST, Wardlaw AJ, Pavord ID, Bradding P: Interleukin-4 and -13 expression is co-localized to mast cells within the airway smooth muscle in asthma. Clin Exp Allergy 2003;33:1711–1716.

20 Gueders MM, Paulissen G, Crahay C, Quesada-Calvo F, Hacha J, Van Hove C, Tournoy K, Louis R, Foidart JM, Noel A, Cataldo DD: Mouse models of asthma: a comparison between C57BL/6 and BALB/c strains regarding bronchial responsiveness, inflammation, and cytokine production. Inflamm Res 2009;58:845–854.

Original Paper

International Archives of Allergy and Immunology

Int Arch Allergy Immunol 2010;152(suppl 1):83–89
DOI: 10.1159/000312131

Published online: June 4, 2010

Differential Activation of Eosinophils by 'Probiotic' *Bifidobacterium bifidum* and 'Pathogenic' *Clostridium difficile*

Koa Hosoki[a] Akiko Nakamura[b] Mizuho Nagao[a] Yukiko Hiraguchi[a]
Reiko Tokuda[a] Hideo Wada[b] Tsutomu Nobori[b] Takao Fujisawa[a]

[a]Institute for Clinical Research and [b]Central Clinical Laboratories, Mie University Hospital, Tsu, Japan

Key Words
Bifidobacterium bifidum · *Clostridium difficile* · Food allergy · Human eosinophils · Inflammatory bowel disease · Probiotics

Abstract
Background: Recent studies suggest that probiotics alleviate pathophysiological processes of allergic diseases and inflammatory bowel diseases, whereas 'non-probiotic' microflora has negative effects. However, the underlying mechanisms are not well known, especially in relation to eosinophils, the major effector cells of these inflammatory diseases. ***Objective:*** To investigate the effects of probiotic *Bifidobacterium bifidum* (BB) on human eosinophil functions compared with pathogenic *Clostridium difficile* (CD). ***Methods:*** Peripheral human eosinophils were cultured with heat-killed BB or CD. FISH-labeled CD and BB were incubated with eosinophils visualized by confocal laser scanning microscopy. Superoxide generation and degranulation of eosinophils were measured with the cytochrome c reduction method and the eosinophil-derived neurotoxin (EDN) release assay, respectively. ***Results:*** Confocal microscopy revealed that Cy3-labeled CD and BB were apparently ingested by eosinophils. Both bacteria induced minimal superoxide generation. However, CD elicited significantly higher EDN release than BB. GM-CSF significantly enhanced EDN release by CD but not by BB. Bacterial-induced EDN release was calcium dependent. ***Conclusion:*** The beneficial effect of probiotic BB might be explained, at least in part, by its ability to decrease EDN release from eosinophils compared with 'pathogenic' CD.

Introduction

Probiotics are defined as live microorganisms that confer a health benefit to the host [1]. Evidence shows that probiotics induce several beneficial host responses by blocking pathogenic effects of invasive bacteria and inhibiting excessive responses in innate immunity, thus supporting intestinal epithelial cell homeostasis [2]. Cross-sectional/prospective cohort studies indicated that allergic children were less often colonized with *Bifidobacterium* than non-allergic children [3–10]. Recent clinical trials have suggested that probiotic bacteria decrease and prevent allergic symptoms, especially in atopic dermatitis

KARGER
Fax +41 61 306 12 34
E-Mail karger@karger.ch
www.karger.com

1018–2438/10/1525–0083$26.00/0

Accessible online at:
www.karger.com/iaa

Correspondence to: Dr. Takao Fujisawa
Institute for Clinical Research, Mie National Hospital
357 Osato-kubotacho, Tsu City, Mie 514-0125 (Japan)
Tel. +81 59 232 2531, Fax +81 59 232 5994
E-Mail fujisawa@mie-m.hosp.go.jp

[11, 12]. Administration of probiotics may also be beneficial for inflammatory bowel disease (IBD) and pouchitis [13–15]. On the other hand, a high incidence of *Clostridium difficile* (CD) infection has been reported in IBD [16–18], and comorbid CD infection can have negative effects on the clinical course of IBD [16, 17, 19]. The proportion of *Clostridium* species was increased in the intestinal microflora of children with allergy compared with healthy non-allergic children [5, 8, 10].

Eosinophils have not only been implicated in the pathogenesis of allergic diseases but also in IBD. Eosinophils accumulated in the intestinal mucosa of IBD patients, and elevated levels of eosinophil-specific chemokines (eotaxin) were observed in the serum and feces of patients with active IBD. The severity of murine experimental colitis decreased by abrogation of eotaxin or by selective deletion of an eosinophil granule protein [20, 21]. Intestinal eosinophils may also play a pivotal role in allergic diseases such as food allergy and atopic dermatitis [22–26]. Certain strains of lactobacilli and bifidobacteria have been reported to affect immune functions through enterocytes, antigen-presenting cells, regulatory T cells, and effector T and B cells [2, 11]. The effects of the intestinal microflora on eosinophil functions are not well understood.

Since numerous eosinophils reside in the intestine both in normal and inflammatory states, we hypothesized that intestinal microbiota may modify the functions of human eosinophils, and consequently play important roles in the pathophysiology of IBD and allergic diseases. Here we examined the effects of probiotic *Bifidobacterium bifidum* (BB) on human eosinophil functions in comparison to CD.

Materials and Methods

Reagents

Percoll was obtained from Pharmacia (Uppsala, Sweden). Anti-CD16 antibody-coated magnetic beads were purchased from Miltenyi Biotec (Anburn, Calif., USA). Hanks' balanced salt solution (HBSS), 4-(2-hydroxyethyl)piperazine-1-ethanesulfonic acid (HEPES) buffer solution and fetal bovine serum (FBS) were obtained from Life Technologies (Grand Island, N.Y., USA). Recombinant human granulocyte-macrophage colony-stimulating factor (GM-CSF) and tumor necrosis factor-α (TNF-α) were from PeproTech (Rocky Hill, N.J., USA). Horse heart ferricytochrome c (type VI), superoxide dismutase (SOD), gelatin, human albumin, RPMI-1640 and ethylene glycol tetraacetic acid (EGTA) were purchased from Sigma-Aldrich (St. Louis, Mo., USA). Pertussis toxin (PTX) was obtained from Calbiochem (San Diego, Calif., USA). The concentrations of these reagents were based on previous studies [27–29].

Preparation of Eosinophils

Eosinophils were purified from healthy adult volunteers with Percoll density gradient centrifugation and negative immunomagnetic bead selection (MACS anti-CD16 microbeads) [30]. The purity of eosinophils was >99.8%.

Preparation of Bacterial Strains

BD (JCM No. 1209, ATCC No. 11863) and CD (JCM No. 1296, ATCC No. 9689) were obtained from the BioResource Center, RIKEN (Tsukuba, Japan). They were incubated at 35°C under anaerobic conditions for approximately 48 h, and centrifuged for 20 min at 3,000 *g*. Subsequently, the bacteria were washed and suspended in PBS and killed by heating at 121°C for 15 min. The processed bacterial strains were stored at –80°C until used for experiments.

Confocal Microscopy

Fluorescence in situ hybridization (FISH) of CD and BB using 16S rRNA-targeted oligonucleotide kits was performed according to the manufacturer's instructions (Ribo Technologies; Groningen, The Netherlands). After washing, FISH-labeled CD and BB were incubated with eosinophils for 1 h at 37°C and 5% CO_2 and visualized using confocal laser scanning microscopy with FluoView software (FV1000; Olympus, Tokyo, Japan). CD and BB were visualized in red with the fluorescence of Cy3. A green light excitation filter (488 nm) was used to detect autofluorescence of eosinophils [31].

Superoxide Anion Generation

Superoxide anion (O_2^-) generation by eosinophils was measured by SOD-induced inhibition of cytochrome c reduction using a modified method reported elsewhere [32]. In brief, freshly purified eosinophils (1.25×10^6 cells/ml) were preincubated at a concentration of 1×10^8 CFU/ml of BB or CD in 96-well tissue culture plates for 30 min at 37°C and 5% CO_2, and resuspended in HBSS with 10 mM HEPES, 0.03% gelatin and 100 μM cytochrome c. Eosinophils in bacterial suspension were dispensed onto the wells of 96-well tissue culture plates, followed by the addition of GM-CSF or TNF-α; reaction was assessed by absorbance at 550 nm over 4 h at 37°C under 5% CO_2 in a microplate autoreader (Wallac 1420 ARVO MX; PerkinElmer, Waltham, Mass., USA). Superoxide anion generation was calculated with an extinction coefficient of $21.1 \times 10^3\ cm^{-1} \times mol^{-1} \times l$ for reduced cytochrome c at 550 nm and was expressed in nanomoles of superoxide produced per 10^5 cells. Each reaction was carried out in duplicate and compared with an identical control reaction that contained 20 μg/ml SOD.

Eosinophil-Derived Neurotoxin

Freshly isolated eosinophils were suspended in RPMI with 10% FBS at 1×10^5 cells/ml and incubated with BB and/or CD at 1×10^8 CFU/ml in 96-well tissue culture plates in the presence or absence of GM-CSF (1 ng/ml) or TNF-α (10 ng/ml) for 4 h at 37°C and 5% CO_2. The cell-free supernatants were collected and stored at –20°C until assayed for EDN using an EDN ELISA kit (MBL, Nagoya, Japan) according to the manufacturer's instructions. Total EDN was determined by lysing eosinophils (1×10^5 cells/ml RPMI with 10% FBS) with an equal volume of polyoxyethylene (9) octylphenyl ether (NP-40). To examine calcium dependency of eosinophil degranulation, cells were preincubated with 1 mM

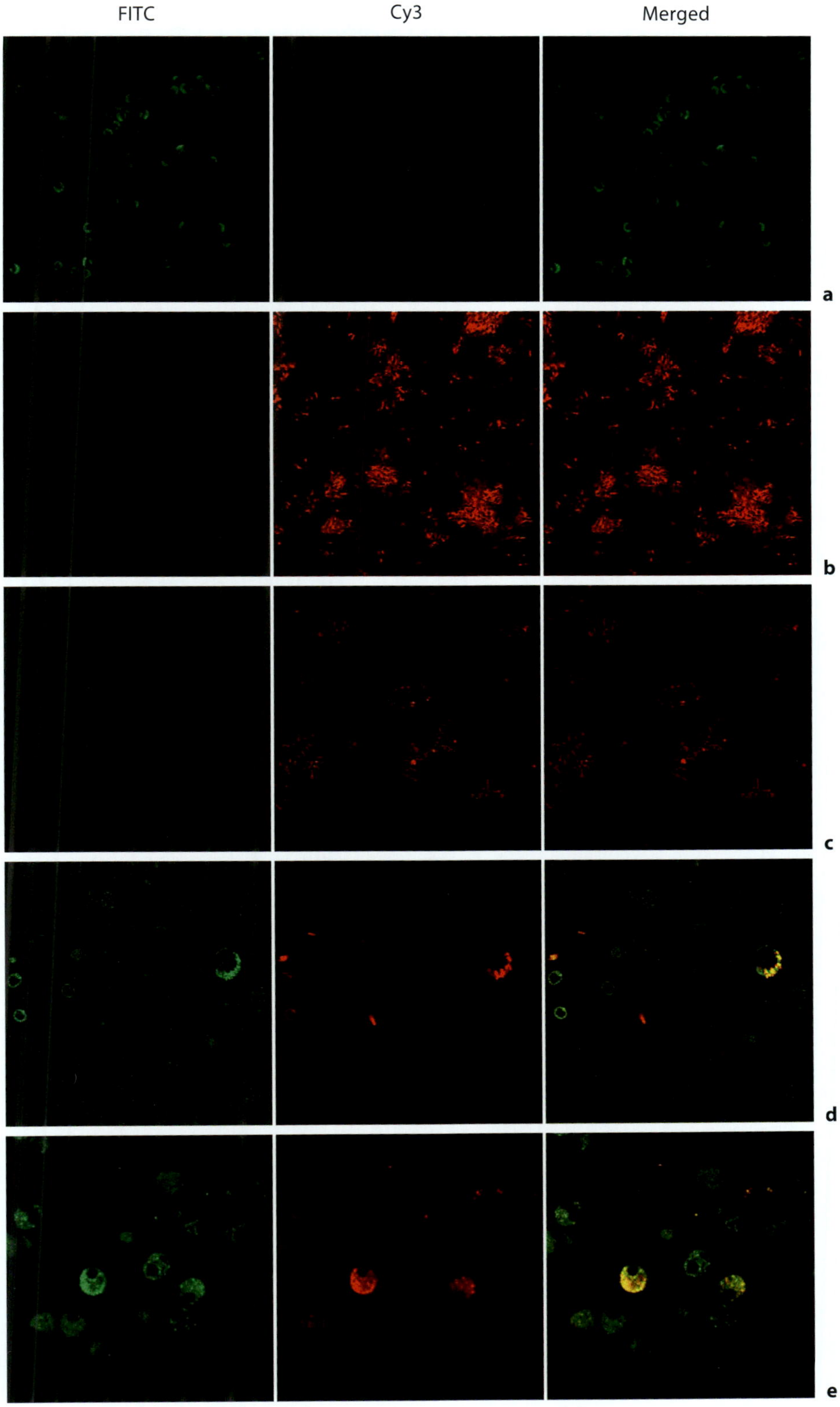

Fig. 1. Imagings of confocal microscopy. **a** Eosinophils. **b** FISH-labeled CD. **c** FISH-labeled BB. **d** Eosinophils co-cultured with FISH-labeled CD. **e** Eosinophils co-cultured with FISH-labeled BD.

EGTA for 15 min at 37°C in 5% CO_2 followed by bacterial stimulation. Preincubation with 100 ng/ml of PTX for 2 h at room temperature was also performed before incubation with bacteria.

Statistical Analysis

Data are expressed as means ± SEM. For multiple-group comparisons, effects of different treatments were analyzed for eosinophils with two-way repeated-measure ANOVA. Significance of individual differences was evaluated using Bonferroni's multiple-comparison tests, if ANOVA was significant.

Results

Confocal Imaging

First, we examined the interaction of eosinophils with bacteria using confocal laser microscopy. After incubation of eosinophils with bacteria for 1 h, Cy3-labeled CD and BB were apparently ingested by eosinophils (fig. 1).

Superoxide Production Assay

Both CD and BB appeared to induce superoxide production from eosinophils, but differences over medium treatment did not reach statistical significance (fig. 2a). GM-CSF enhanced superoxide generation but again both bacteria had minimal effect (fig. 2b).

EDN Release Assay

Both CD- and BB-induced degranulation was assessed by EDN release from eosinophils. CD-induced degranulation was significantly higher than that induced by BB (fig. 3a). EDN release from eosinophils co-cultured with CD were blocked by pretreatment with EGTA, indicating that bacterial-induced EDN release was an active process dependent on intracellular Ca^{2+} signaling. PTX did not have any effect on CD- or BB-induced degranulation, indicating that bacterial-induced EDN release was independent of G-protein signaling (fig. 3b). Enhancement of the degranulation by GM-CSF or TNF-α was observed only in CD- but not BB-induced reactions, and there was a statistically significant enhancement by GM-CSF in CD-induced reactions (fig. 3c). We also tested whether bacterial culture supernatant or simple latex beads induced EDN or cytokine release using the above-described protocol. The culture supernatant and latex beads did not have any effect on human eosinophils (data not shown), indicating that direct, specific interactions with bacteria, possibly through phagocytosis, caused eosinophil degranulation. EDN release from eosinophils incubated with BB and/or CD at 1×10^6 CFU/ml and 1×10^7 CFU/ml was not significantly different.

Discussion

The intestinal microflora has been implicated in the pathophysiology of allergy and IBD, although the mechanisms of action have not been elucidated [11–15]. Eosinophil infiltration into the intestinal mucosa is a pathological hallmark of the disease. The present study revealed that EDN release induced by probiotic BB was significantly lower than that by CD, even in the presence of eosinophil-activating cytokines. These results suggested that the differential responses of eosinophils to probiotic and pathogenic bacteria may in part explain the pathogenesis of eosinophil-related intestinal diseases.

In intestinal biopsy specimens, eosinophil degranulation was significantly increased in patients with cow-milk-sensitive enteropathy compared with normal controls [33, 34]. Patients with food allergy also demonstrated higher fecal concentrations of eosinophil granule products than healthy controls [22, 23, 35]. Evidence of eosinophil degranulation was often seen in the mucosa, feces and gut lavage fluid in IBD [36–39]. Eosinophil degranulation was able to damage the gastrointestinal mucosal barrier. It has been reported that the epithelial barrier function of T84 cells was significantly impaired when basolateral surfaces were exposed to native human major basic protein [40]. The present study demonstrated that CD induced significantly higher eosinophil degranulation, suggesting that CD may possibly enhance intestinal permeability. Increased absorption of food allergen due to gut barrier dysfunction caused by excessive eosinophil degranulation may explain why infants who have predominantly CD in their intestinal flora have food allergy. In addition, CD infection increases disease activity and mortality in IBD patients [16, 41].

We showed that eosinophil degranulation by CD requires at least intracellular Ca signaling. CD-induced degranulation was not dependent on PTX-sensitive G proteins. Intracellular signaling of the CD-induced reaction warrants further investigation.

A limitation of our study may be that a direct contact between eosinophils and bacteria, especially probiotics, may not occur in vivo, and thus our experimental condition would be unrealistic. In healthy subjects, most eosinophils reside in the lamina propria in the stomach and intestine [42, 43]. However, infiltrating eosinophils were observed throughout the reticular connective tissue of the lamina propria and mucosa, and throughout the length of the lamina propria of the villi in oral allergen-

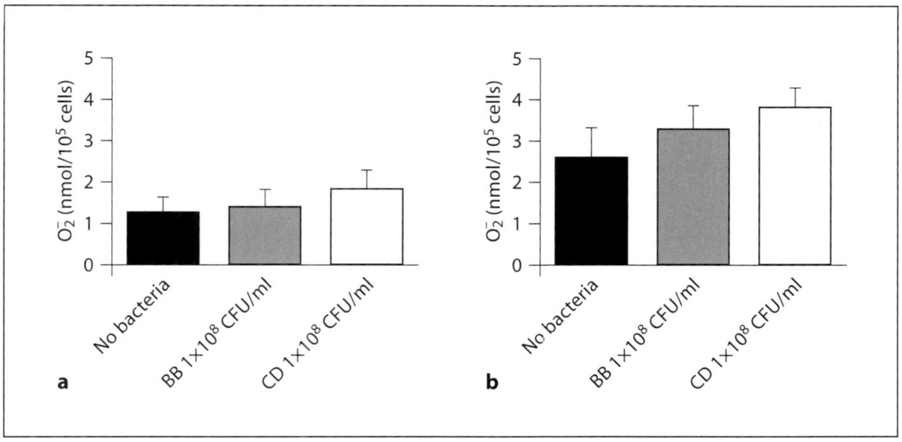

Fig. 2. Superoxide generation by eosinophils co-cultured with BB or CD in the absence (**a**) and presence of GM-CSF (1 ng/ml; **b**) measured by SOD-inhibitable reduction of cytochrome c. The reactions were measured for absorbance at 550 nm over 4 h in a microplate autoreader. Superoxide anion generation was calculated with an extinction coefficient of 21.1 × 10^3 cm^{-1} × mol^{-1} × l for reduced cytochrome c at 550 nm and was expressed in nanomoles of superoxide produced per 10^5 cells. Means ± SEM (n = 4).

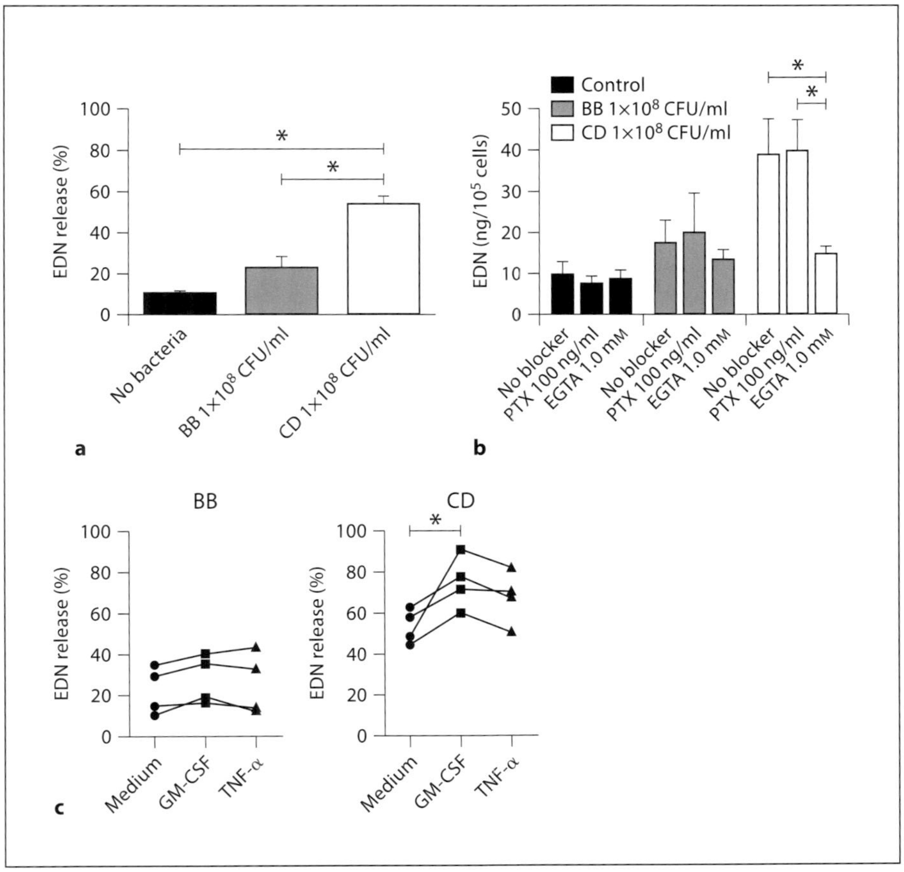

Fig. 3. EDN release induced by BB and CD (* $p < 0.05$, n = 4). Eosinophils were incubated with BB and/or CD at 1 × 10^8 CFU/ml in 96-well tissue culture plates in the presence or absence of GM-CSF (1 ng/ml) or TNF-α (10 ng/ml) for 4 h at 37°C and 5% CO_2. The cell-free supernatants were collected and stored at –20°C until assayed for EDN with an ELISA kit. Total EDN was determined by lysing eosinophils (1 × 10^5cells/ml RPMI with 10% FBS) with an equal volume of polyoxyethylene (9) octylphenyl ether (NP-40). **a** Percent EDN release induced by BB or CD. **b** Net EDN release from eosinophils preincubated with medium alone, PTX (100 ng/ml) and EGTA (1.0 mM) before co-culture with bacteria. **c** Piecemeal percent EDN release induced by BB and CD in the presence or absence of eosinophil-activating cytokines, GM-CSF (1 ng/ml) and TNF-α (10 ng/ml).

challenged mice [44]. Furthermore, eosinophil-specific markers were recognized in stool samples of food-allergic and IBD patients [20, 22, 23, 34, 35, 45]. Consequently, we hypothesize that a direct interaction between eosinophils and gut flora may occur during pathological conditions.

In conclusion, we show that BB induces significantly less EDN release from eosinophils than CD. The results may explain, at least in part, the pathophysiological involvement of intestinal microbiota through eosinophils in the intestine in allergy and IBD.

Acknowledgments

This work was supported by a Grant-in-Aid for Scientific Research from the Ministry of Health, Labor and Welfare of Japan. We thank Ms. Manami Negoro and Ms. Kyoko Nishinaka for their excellent technical assistance.

Disclosure Statement

The authors declare that no financial or other conflict of interest exists in relation to the content of this article.

References

1 Sanders ME: Probiotics: considerations for human health. Nutr Rev 2003;61:91–99.

2 Vanderpool C, Yan F, Polk DB: Mechanisms of probiotic action: implications for therapeutic applications in inflammatory bowel diseases. Inflamm Bowel Dis 2008;14:1585–1596.

3 Suzuki S, Shimojo N, Tajiri Y, Kumemura M, Kohno Y: Differences in the composition of intestinal Bifidobacterium species and the development of allergic diseases in infants in rural Japan. Clin Exp Allergy 2007;37:506–511.

4 Bjorksten B, Naaber P, Sepp E, Mikelsaar M: The intestinal microflora in allergic Estonian and Swedish 2-year-old children. Clin Exp Allergy 1999;29:342–346.

5 Sepp E, Julge K, Mikelsaar M, Bjorksten B: Intestinal microbiota and immunoglobulin E responses in 5-year-old Estonian children. Clin Exp Allergy 2005;35:1141–1146.

6 Murray CS, Tannock GW, Simon MA, Harmsen HJ, Welling GW, Custovic A, Woodcock A: Fecal microbiota in sensitized wheezy and non-sensitized non-wheezy children: a nested case-control study. Clin Exp Allergy 2005;35:741–745.

7 Watanabe S, Narisawa Y, Arase S, Okamatsu H, Ikenaga T, Tajiri Y, Kumemura M: Differences in fecal microflora between patients with atopic dermatitis and healthy control subjects. J Allergy Clin Immunol 2003;111:587–591.

8 Bjorksten B, Sepp E, Julge K, Voor T, Mikelsaar M: Allergy development and the intestinal microflora during the first year of life. J Allergy Clin Immunol 2001;108:516–520.

9 Ouwehand AC, Isolauri E, He F, Hashimoto H, Benno Y, Salminen S: Differences in Bifidobacterium flora composition in allergic and healthy infants. J Allergy Clin Immunol 2001;108:144–145.

10 Kalliomaki M, Kirjavainen P, Eerola E, Kero P, Salminen S, Isolauri E: Distinct patterns of neonatal gut microflora in infants in whom atopy was and was not developing. J Allergy Clin Immunol 2001;107:129–134.

11 Prescott SL, Bjorksten B: Probiotics for the prevention or treatment of allergic diseases. J Allergy Clin Immunol 2007;120:255–262.

12 Lee J, Seto D, Bielory L: Meta-analysis of clinical trials of probiotics for prevention and treatment of pediatric atopic dermatitis. J Allergy Clin Immunol 2008;121:116–121e111.

13 Ewaschuk JB, Dieleman LA: Probiotics and prebiotics in chronic inflammatory bowel diseases. World J Gastroenterol 2006;12:5941–5950.

14 Isaacs K, Herfarth H: Role of probiotic therapy in IBD. Inflamm Bowel Dis 2008;14:1597–1605.

15 Hedin C, Whelan K, Lindsay JO: Evidence for the use of probiotics and prebiotics in inflammatory bowel disease: a review of clinical trials. Proc Nutr Soc 2007;66:307–315.

16 Nguyen GC, Kaplan GG, Harris ML, Brant SR: A national survey of the prevalence and impact of *Clostridium difficile* infection among hospitalized inflammatory bowel disease patients. Am J Gastroenterol 2008;103:1443–1450.

17 Issa M, Vijayapal A, Graham MB, Beaulieu DB, Otterson MF, Lundeen S, Skaros S, Weber LR, Komorowski RA, Knox JF, Emmons J, Bajaj JS, Binion DG: Impact of *Clostridium difficile* on inflammatory bowel disease. Clin Gastroenterol Hepatol 2007;5:345–351.

18 Rodemann JF, Dubberke ER, Reske KA, Seo da H, Stone CD: Incidence of *Clostridium difficile* infection in inflammatory bowel disease. Clin Gastroenterol Hepatol 2007;5:339–344.

19 Freeman HJ: Recent developments on the role of *Clostridium difficile* in inflammatory bowel disease. World J Gastroenterol 2008;14:2794–2796.

20 Wedemeyer J, Vosskuhl K: Role of gastrointestinal eosinophils in inflammatory bowel disease and intestinal tumours. Best Pract Res Clin Gastroenterol 2008;22:537–549.

21 Carvalho AT, Elia CC, de Souza HS, Elias PR, Pontes EL, Lukashok HP, de Freitas FC, Lapa e Silva JR: Immunohistochemical study of intestinal eosinophils in inflammatory bowel disease. J Clin Gastroenterol 2003;36:120–125.

22 Majamaa H, Laine S, Miettinen A: Eosinophil protein X and eosinophil cationic protein as indicators of intestinal inflammation in infants with atopic eczema and food allergy. Clin Exp Allergy 1999;29:1502–1506.

23 Majamaa H, Miettinen A, Laine S, Isolauri E: Intestinal inflammation in children with atopic eczema: faecal eosinophil cationic protein and tumour necrosis factor-alpha as non-invasive indicators of food allergy. Clin Exp Allergy 1996;26:181–187.

24 Schwab D, Muller S, Aigner T, Neureiter D, Kirchner T, Hahn EG, Raithel M: Functional and morphologic characterization of eosinophils in the lower intestinal mucosa of patients with food allergy. Am J Gastroenterol 2003;98:1525–1534.

25 Kosnai I, Kuitunen P, Savilahti E, Sipponen P: Mast cells and eosinophils in the jejunal mucosa of patients with intestinal cow's milk allergy and celiac disease of childhood. J Pediatr Gastroenterol Nutr 1984;3:368–372.

26 Rothenberg ME: Eosinophilic gastrointestinal disorders (EGID). J Allergy Clin Immunol 2004;113:11–28, quiz 29.

27 Inoue Y, Matsuwaki Y, Shin SH, Ponikau JU, Kita H: Nonpathogenic, environmental fungi induce activation and degranulation of human eosinophils. J Immunol 2005;175:5439–5447.

28 Takeuchi M, Tatsumi Y, Kitaichi K, Baba K, Suzuki R, Shibata E, Takagi K, Miyamoto K, Hasegawa T: Selective phosphodiesterase type 4 inhibitors reduce the prolonged survival of eosinophils stimulated by granulocyte-macrophage colony-stimulating factor. Biol Pharm Bull 2002;25:184–187.

29 Horie S, Gleich GJ, Kita H: Cytokines directly induce degranulation and superoxide production from human eosinophils. J Allergy Clin Immunol 1996;98:371–381.

30 Fujisawa T, Kato Y, Nagase H, Atsuta J, Terada A, Iguchi K, Kamiya H, Morita Y, Kitaura M, Kawasaki H, Yoshie O, Hirai K: Chemokines induce eosinophil degranulation through CCR-3. J Allergy Clin Immunol 2000;106:507–513.

31 Weil GJ, Chused TM: Eosinophil autofluorescence and its use in isolation and analysis of human eosinophils using flow microfluorometry. Blood 1981;57:1099–1104.

32 Nagata M, Sedgwick JB, Kita H, Busse WW: Granulocyte macrophage colony-stimulating factor augments ICAM-1 and VCAM-1 activation of eosinophil function. Am J Respir Cell Mol Biol 1998;19:158–166.

33 Chung HL, Hwang JB, Kwon YD, Park MH, Shin WJ, Park JB: Deposition of eosinophil-granule major basic protein and expression of intercellular adhesion molecule-1 and vascular cell adhesion molecule-1 in the mucosa of the small intestine in infants with cow's milk-sensitive enteropathy. J Allergy Clin Immunol 1999;103:1195–1201.

34 Bengtsson U, Knutson TW, Knutson L, Dannaeus A, Hallgren R, Ahlstedt S: Eosinophil cationic protein and histamine after intestinal challenge in patients with cow's milk intolerance. J Allergy Clin Immunol 1997;100: 216–221.
35 Saarinen KM, Sarnesto A, Savilahti E: Markers of inflammation in the feces of infants with cow's milk allergy. Pediatr Allergy Immunol 2002;13:188–194.
36 Raab Y, Fredens K, Gerdin B, Hallgren R: Eosinophil activation in ulcerative colitis: studies on mucosal release and localization of eosinophil granule constituents. Dig Dis Sci 1998;43:1061–1070.
37 Peterson CG, Sangfelt P, Wagner M, Hansson T, Lettesjo H, Carlson M: Fecal levels of leukocyte markers reflect disease activity in patients with ulcerative colitis. Scand J Clin Lab Invest 2007;67:810–820.
38 Carlson M, Raab Y, Peterson C, Hallgren R, Venge P: Increased intraluminal release of eosinophil granule proteins EPO, ECP, EPX, and cytokines in ulcerative colitis and proctitis in segmental perfusion. Am J Gastroenterol 1999;94:1876–1883.
39 Levy AM, Gleich GJ, Sandborn WJ, Tremaine WJ, Steiner BL, Phillips SF: Increased eosinophil granule proteins in gut lavage fluid from patients with inflammatory bowel disease. Mayo Clin Proc 1997;72:117–123.
40 Furuta GT, Nieuwenhuis EE, Karhausen J, Gleich G, Blumberg RS, Lee JJ, Ackerman SJ: Eosinophils alter colonic epithelial barrier function: role for major basic protein. Am J Physiol Gastrointest Liver Physiol 2005; 289:G890–G897.
41 Pascarella F, Martinelli M, Miele E, Pezzo MD, Roscetto E, Staiano A: Impact of *Clostridium difficile* infection on pediatric inflammatory bowel disease. J Pediatr 2009; 154:854–858.
42 Matthews AN, Friend DS, Zimmermann N, Sarafi MN, Luster AD, Pearlman E, Wert SE, Rothenberg ME: Eotaxin is required for the baseline level of tissue eosinophils. Proc Natl Acad Sci USA 1998;95:6273–6278.
43 Furuta GT: Emerging questions regarding eosinophil's role in the esophago-gastrointestinal tract. Curr Opin Gastroenterol 2006; 22:658–663.
44 Hogan SP, Mishra A, Brandt EB, Foster PS, Rothenberg ME: A critical role for eotaxin in experimental oral antigen-induced eosinophilic gastrointestinal allergy. Proc Natl Acad Sci USA 2000;97:6681–6686.
45 Bischoff SC, Grabowsky J, Manns MP: Quantification of inflammatory mediators in stool samples of patients with inflammatory bowel disorders and controls. Dig Dis Sci 1997;42:394–403.

Review

International Archives of Allergy and Immunology

Int Arch Allergy Immunol 2010;152(suppl 1):90–95
DOI: 10.1159/000312132

Published online: June 4, 2010

The Pathophysiological Roles of PI3Ks and Therapeutic Potential of Selective Inhibitors in Allergic Inflammation

Masahide Takeda[a] Wataru Ito[a] Masako Tanabe[a] Shigeharu Ueki[a] Junko Kihara[a] Hikari Kato[a] Tomomi Tanigai[a] Hiroyuki Kayaba[a] Takehiko Sasaki[b] Junichi Chihara[a]

Departments of [a]Infection, Allergy, Clinical Immunology and Laboratory Medicine, and [b]Pathology and Immunology, Akita University Graduate School of Medicine, Akita, Japan

Key Words

Airway inflammation · Allergy · Asthma · Phosphoinositide 3-kinase · PI3K inhibitors

Abstract

Phosphoinositide 3-kinases (PI3Ks) are known to be involved in a variety of cellular responses such as cell survival, proliferation, differentiation and cell migration. Recently, PI3Ks have been associated with the pathogenesis of asthma because various immune cells regulate allergic responses. Among the three classes of PI3Ks, the roles of PI3Kγ and PI3Kδ in allergic responses have attracted particular attention. In a previous report, allergic airway hyperresponsiveness (AHR), inflammation and airway remodeling in an ovalbumin-induced asthma model were decreased in PI3Kγ-deficient mice compared with wild-type mice. In addition, AHR and inflammation were attenuated by administration of a selective PI3Kδ inhibitor in a murine model of asthma. These results indicate that PI3Kγ and PI3Kδ may be new therapeutic targets for asthma. However, PI3Kγ and PI3Kδ may differ in terms of the mechanism of regulation. In this review, we focus on the roles of PI3Kγ and PI3Kδ in the pathogenesis of asthma and discuss the mechanistic differences between PI3Kγ and PI3Kδ.

Introduction

Phosphoinositide 3-kinases (PI3Ks) are a family of proteins that phosphorylate the 3′-OH position of the inositol ring of phosphatidylinositols, which are located in the cellular membrane, resulting in the formation of phosphoinositide (3,4,5) triphosphate. PI3Ks play a prominent role in all eukaryotic cellular responses, including cell survival, proliferation, differentiation and cell migration because phosphoinositide (3,4,5) triphosphate activates various downstream signaling pathways [1]. Therefore, PI3Ks are thought to be involved in the pathogenesis of a variety of diseases such as cancer, inflammation and allergy.

PI3Ks can be divided into three classes: class I, II and III [2]. Class I PI3Ks have attracted particular attention since these enzymes are activated upon receptor stimulation. The class IA PI3Ks are activated by stimulation of tyrosine kinase-based receptors and consist of a heterodimeric complex composed of a 110-kDa (p110α, p110β and p110δ) catalytic subunit and adaptor proteins (p85α and p85β and p55α, p55β and p55γ). PI3Kγ, the only member of class IB, is found to be activated by stimulation of βγ subunits of G protein-coupled receptor and consists of a heterodimer composed of p110γ and p101 adaptor pro-

KARGER

Fax +41 61 306 12 34
E-Mail karger@karger.ch
www.karger.com

1018–2438/10/1525–0090$26.00/0

Accessible online at:
www.karger.com/iaa

Correspondence to: Dr. Junichi Chihara
Department of Infection, Allergy, Clinical Immunology and Laboratory Medicine
Akita University Graduate School of Medicine
1-1-1, Hondo, Akita 010-8543 (Japan)
Tel. +81 18 884 6180, Fax +81 18 836 2624, E-Mail chihara@hos.akita-u.ac.jp

teins. Recently, the focus has been on the relationship between PI3Ks and asthma because various immune cells are implicated in the pathogenesis of asthma [3, 4]. In fact, it has already been reported that acute asthmatic responses in a murine model were diminished by administration of LY294002, a pharmacological inhibitor of PI3K [5, 6]. However, pan-PI3K inhibitors, such as LY294002, may be highly toxic to the body because fetal death has been reported in PI3Kα- and PI3Kβ-deficient mice [7, 8]. Therefore, involvement of PI3K isoforms in asthma has recently received attention. In this paper, we focus on the association between PI3K isoforms and the pathogenesis of asthma.

Effect of PI3K in a Murine Model of Asthma

Some researchers have investigated the role of PI3Ks in experimental asthma models. Regarding class IA PI3K, Lee et al. [9] showed that intratracheal instillation of IC87114, a selective p110δ inhibitor, significantly attenuated allergic airway inflammation and airway hyperresponsiveness (AHR) as well as Th2 cytokine production in a murine model of asthma. Furthermore, it was demonstrated that these allergic responses were decreased in ovalbumin (OVA)-sensitized and -challenged p110δ mutant mice [10]. These results indicate that PI3Kδ is implicated in asthma and may be a therapeutic target of asthma.

On the other hand, we investigated the role of PI3Kγ in the pathogenesis of asthma using PI3Kγ-deficient mice, and we showed that allergic AHR, airway inflammation as well as Th2 cytokine production in bronchoalveolar lavage fluid were significantly decreased in a PI3Kγ-deficient asthma model compared with the wild type (WT) [11]. In contrast to PI3Kδ and PI3Kγ, we cannot investigate the association of PI3Kα and PI3Kβ in experimental asthma because of fetal death in PI3Kα- and PI3Kβ-deficient mice. In addition, there are few experimental reports demonstrating the role of PI3Kα and PI3Kβ using these selective inhibitors. Therefore, we focus on the effect of PI3Kγ and PI3Kδ on asthma in the next part.

PI3Kγ Regulates Airway Remodeling

Even now there are some patients laden with severe asthma. Therefore, how to manage severe asthma is a challenge in asthma care. Involvement of irreversible airway change, i.e. airway remodeling, is indicated as a factor in severe asthma [12]. Therefore, molecules that regulate airway remodeling are thought to be new therapeutic targets for asthma. Although airway remodeling is difficult to define, subepithelial fibrosis, goblet cell hyperplasia and myofibroblast hypertrophy due to chronic airway inflammation have been identified as components of this response [12, 13]. We also investigated the association of PI3Kγ with airway remodeling using histological staining of lung tissue, which revealed that the histological features of airway remodeling were decreased in a PI3Kγ-deficient asthma model [11]. On the other hand, the role of PI3Kδ in airway remodeling needs further examination because there have been few investigations of the relationship between PI3Kδ and airway remodeling except for a study that showed that IC87114 attenuated mucus production expressed as PAS-positive staining in OVA-induced asthma [9]. These results may lead to the assumption that PI3Kγ may be a new therapeutic target of severe asthma.

Lack of an Effect of PI3Kγ in OVA-Specific IgE Production

It is known that immunological responses such as IgE production, alterations in T-cell phenotype and the shift in the Th1/Th2 balance occur in bronchial asthma [14, 15]. In our study, there was no significant difference in serum OVA-specific IgE and IgG1 or the percentage of CD3+CD4+ T cells in bronchoalveolar lavage fluid between OVA-sensitized and -challenged (OVA/OVA) PI3Kγ-deficient and WT mice. These results suggest that PI3Kγ may have no effect on the T-cell phenotype, Th1/Th2 balance and IgE production in bronchial asthma. Therefore, the results in our study may indicate that the observed reduction in AHR, airway inflammation and airway remodeling in OVA/OVA PI3Kγ-deficient mice may be caused by regulation in the challenge/effector phase of asthma but not in the induction phase.

To determine in which phase of the allergic response PI3Kγ plays a vital role, we transferred splenocytes from OVA-sensitized WT or PI3Kγ-deficient mice to respective naïve mice. As a result, inflammatory cell infiltration into the airways was detected in both WT recipient mice but not in PI3Kγ-deficient recipient mice [11]. We also investigated inflammatory cell infiltration into airway tissue by means of histological examination using hematoxylin-eosin staining. Similarly, inflammatory cell infiltration was detected in both WT recipient mice. Moreover, methacholine dose-dependently increased AHR in both

WT recipient mice ($p < 0.05$; fig. 1). These results indicate that PI3Kγ is involved in the pathogenesis of asthma via modulation of the challenge/effector phase of asthma.

There are several possible reasons why inflammatory cell infiltration was detected in both WT recipient mice. One is a decrease in chemokine production from fibroblasts and epithelial cells. Another is a decrease in the ability to adhere to endothelial cells. The last possibility is a decrease in the chemotactic activity of inflammatory cells in PI3Kγ-deficient mice. Lim et al. [16] reported that there was no significant difference between WT and PI3Kγ asthma models at the level of lung tissue eotaxin-1. In addition, Pinho et al. [17] demonstrated that eosinophils from PI3Kγ-deficient mice have weaker chemotactic activity compared to WT eosinophils using an experimental allergic inflammation model. They also showed that the presence of PI3Kγ in eosinophils was important for migration in experiments with chimeric mice. These results suggest that PI3Kγ in eosinophils plays an important role in the chemotaxis of eosinophils into airway tissue but not PI3Kγ in parenchymal cells.

On the other hand, it was reported that OVA-specific IgE was attenuated by a PI3Kδ inhibitor. Class IA PI3Ks are known to be implicated in early B-cell development and B-cell function [18, 19]. These results support the notion that PI3Kδ is associated with IgE production. Moreover, in the case of adoptive splenocyte transfer using PI3Kδ mutant mice, an increase in eosinophils in bronchoalveolar lavage fluid was detected only when splenocytes from WT mice were transferred, which is contrary to our results [10]. These results indicate that PI3Kδ is involved in the pathogenesis of asthma through a mechanism that differs from that of PI3Kγ, especially regulating the induction phase of asthma. However, the detailed mechanism is still unclear. Therefore further studies are necessary to elucidate the mechanism behind this difference between PI3Kγ and PI3Kδ in terms of allergic responses.

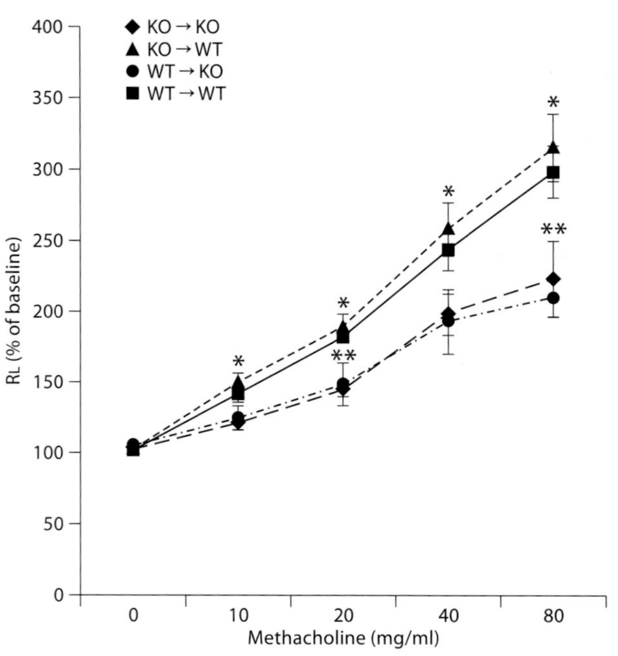

Fig. 1. Lung resistance (RL) to increasing methacholine doses was significantly increased in both WT recipient mice (measured using an invasive system from Sigma-Aldrich, as previously described [28]). Once baseline data were established, saline and increasing doses of nebulized methacholine were administered. In each dose, airflow changes in the sealed chamber and pressure changes in the airways were analyzed using BioSystem XA software (Buxco Electronics) for 3 min. Pulmonary resistance was expressed as a percent change from baseline. Results for each group are expressed as the mean ± SD. * $p < 0.05$, PI3Kγ-deficient splenocytes to PI3Kγ-deficient naïve mice vs. PI3Kγ-deficient splenocytes to WT naïve mice. ** $p < 0.05$, PI3Kγ-deficient splenocytes to PI3Kγ-deficient naïve mice vs. WT splenocytes to WT naïve mice. KO = Knockout.

Role of PI3K Isoforms in Other Immune Cells

The roles of PI3Ks in other immune cells have also been studied. For example, Salogni et al. [20] demonstrated that dendritic cell migration to CCL3 and activin A was decreased in PI3Kγ-deficient mice. Del Prete et al. [21] also reported that dendritic cells from PI3Kγ-deficient mice had a reduced ability to respond to chemokines and exhibited less activity in terms of the antigen-presenting response than WT mice. Mast cells also play an important role in allergic responses. Cytokine production and degranulation, in particular, are crucial. Ali et al. [22] confirmed that IC87114 suppressed cytokine production and degranulation from mast cells. They also described the superiority of PI3Kδ for the regulation of mast cell function in vivo although they demonstrated that PI3Kγ and PI3Kδ play an important role in FcεRI-activated mast cell degranulation in vitro [23]. On the other hand, Endo et al. [24] reported that AS605240, a selective inhibitor of PI3Kγ, inhibited degranulation of bone marrow-derived mast cells. Neutrophils are also associated with asthma, especially steroid-resistant asthma, because neutrophils are likely to be detected in the airway tissue of steroid-resistant asthma patients. Sasaki

Table 1. Summary of the role of PI3Kγ and PI3Kδ in the pathogenesis of asthma and asthma-related immune cell functions

	Experimental model/cell type	Effects		References
In vivo				
PI3Kγ-deficient mice	OVA-induced asthma model	decrease of:	AHR airway inflammation Th2 cytokine production airway remodeling	11
		no influence on:	IgE production	
PI3Kγ-deficient mice	OVA-induced asthma model	decrease of:	airway inflammation	29
		no influence on:	IgE production	
		regulate eosinophil migration		
PI3Kγ-deficient mice	OVA-induced asthma model	decrease of:	AHR airway inflammation airway remodeling	16
		no influence on:	chemokine production	
	OVA-induced asthma model	decrease of:	AHR airway inflammation Th2 cytokine production	10
IC87114 (PI3Kδ inhibitor)	OVA-induced asthma model	attenuation of:	AHR airway inflammation PAS-positive cells Th2 cytokine production chemokine production IgE production	9
TG100-115 (PI3Kγ/PI3Kδ inhibitor)	OVA-induced asthma model	attenuation of:	AHR airway inflammation	27
In vitro				
AS605240 (PI3Kγ inhibitor)	mast cells	attenuation of:	degranulation	23
AS605240	mast cells	attenuation of:	migration degranulation	24
PI3Kγ-deficient mice	eosinophils	decrease of:	migration	17
PI3Kγ-deficient mice	dendritic cells	decrease of:	migration	20
PI3Kγ-deficient mice	dendritic cells	decrease of:	migration antigen-presenting response	21
IC87114	mast cells	attenuation of:	degranulation cytokine release	22
IC87114	mast cells	attenuation of:	degranulation adhesion	23
PI3Kγ-deficient mice	neutrophils	decrease of:	migration	25

PI3Kγ and PI3Kδ have previously been shown to be involved in allergic responses in asthma using experimental asthma models. In addition, PI3Kγ and PI3Kδ are reported to regulate a variety of asthma-related immune cell functions.

et al. [25] showed that migration of neutrophils from PI3Kγ-deficient mice was decreased compared with WT mice. In addition, Randis et al. [26] demonstrated that PI3Kγ and PI3Kδ play a crucial role in neutrophil migration and neutrophil-induced arthritis using PI3Kγ- and PI3Kδ-deficient mice. In their report, double deletion of PI3Kγ and PI3Kδ had a stronger effect on neutrophil migration and arthritis treatment using PI3Kγ-/PI3Kδ-deficient mice or a combination of PI3Kγ-deficient mice and IC87114. In a mouse model, allergic AHR and inflammation were attenuated by administration of aerosolized TG100-115, a PI3Kγ/PI3Kδ inhibitor [27]. These reports support the possibility that PI3Kγ- and PI3Kδ-selective inhibitors or PI3Kγ/PI3Kδ inhibitors may have therapeutic potential for asthma and other allergic diseases. The effects of PI3K isoforms on asthma and immune cells are summarized in table 1.

Conclusion

Treatment of severe asthma resistant to steroids and of airway remodeling has recently become the subject of asthma management research. Therefore, molecules that regulate allergic responses, including airway remodeling, and have a mechanism of action different from that of steroids might become new therapeutic targets for asthma. PI3Kγ and PI3Kδ reportedly regulate allergic responses, including airway remodeling, and therefore they may become effective therapeutic targets for asthma. Indeed, selective PI3Kγ and PI3Kδ inhibitors had anti-allergic effects in past fundamental research using murine models of asthma and a variety of immune cells. These results lead to the assumption that selective PI3Kγ and PI3Kδ inhibitors may have therapeutic potential for allergic inflammation. On the other hand, it is very interesting that there may be some mechanical differences between PI3Kγ and PI3Kδ. Further studies are needed to identify the detailed mechanisms of action of PI3Kγ and PI3Kδ in asthma to be able to use their selective inhibitors in asthma treatment.

Disclosure Statement

The authors declare that no financial or other conflict of interest exists in relation to the content of this article.

References

1 Toker A, Cantley LC: Signalling through the lipid products of phosphoinositide-3-OH kinase. Nature 1997;387:673–676.
2 Wymann MP, Björklöf K, Calvez R, Finan P, Thomast M, Trifilieff A, Barbier M, Altruda F, Hirsch E, Laffargue M: Phosphoinositide 3-kinase gamma: a key modulator in inflammation and allergy. Biochem Soc Trans 2003; 31:275–280.
3 Chihara J: Molecular mechanisms of eosinophil activation in allergic diseases. Clin Exp All Rev 2005;5:46–49.
4 Larché M, Robinson DS, Kay AB: The role of T lymphocytes in the pathogenesis of asthma. J Allergy Clin Immunol 2003;111:450–463.
5 Duan W, Aguinaldo Datiles AM, Leung BP, Vlahos CJ, Wong WS: An anti-inflammatory role for a phosphoinositide 3-kinase inhibitor LY294002 in a mouse asthma model. Int Immunopharmacol 2005;5:495–502.
6 Kwak YG, Song CH, Yi HK, Hwang PH, Kim JS, Lee KS, Lee YC: Involvement of PTEN in airway hyperresponsiveness and inflammation in bronchial asthma. J Clin Invest 2003; 111:1083–1092.
7 Bi L, Okabe I, Bernard DJ, Wynshaw-Boris A, Nussbaum RL: Proliferative defect and embryonic lethality in mice homozygous for a deletion in the p110alpha subunit of phosphoinositide 3-kinase. J Biol Chem 1999;274: 10963–10968.
8 Bi L, Okabe I, Bernard DJ, Nussbaum RL: Early embryonic lethality in mice deficient in the p110beta catalytic subunit of PI 3-kinase. Mamm Genome 2002;13:169–172.
9 Lee KS, Lee HK, Hayflick JS, Lee YC, Puri KD: Inhibition of phosphoinositide 3-kinase delta attenuates allergic airway inflammation and hyperresponsiveness in murine asthma model. FASEB J 2006;20:455–465.
10 Nashed BF, Zhang T, Al-Alwan M, Srinivasan G, Halayko AJ, Okkenhaug K, Vanhaesebroeck B, Hayglass KT, Marshall AJ: Role of the phosphoinositide 3-kinase p110delta in generation of type 2 cytokine responses and allergic airway inflammation. Eur J Immunol 2007;37:416–424.
11 Takeda M, Ito W, Tanabe M, Ueki S, Kato H, Kihara J, Tanigai T, Chiba T, Yamaguchi K, Kayaba H, Imai Y, Okuyama K, Ohno I, Sasaki T, Chihara J: Allergic airway hyperresponsiveness, inflammation, and remodeling do not develop in phosphoinositide 3-kinase gamma-deficient mice. J Allergy Clin Immunol 2009;123:805–812.
12 Davies DE, Wicks J, Powell RM, Puddicombe SM, Holgate ST: Airway remodeling in asthma: new insights. J Allergy Clin Immunol 2003;111:215–225.
13 Ito W, Kanehiro A, Matsumoto K, Hirano A, Ono K, Maruyama H, Kataoka M, Nakamura T, Gelfand EW, Tanimoto M: Hepatocyte growth factor attenuates airway hyperresponsiveness, inflammation, and remodeling. Am J Respir Cell Mol Biol 2005;32:268–280.
14 Georas SN, Guo J, De Fanis U, Casolaro V: T-helper cell type-2 regulation in allergic disease. Eur Respir J 2005;26:1119–1137.
15 Platts-Mills TA: The role of immunoglobulin E in allergy and asthma. Am J Respir Crit Care Med 2001;164:1–5.
16 Lim DH, Cho JY, Song DJ, Lee SY, Miller M, Broide DH: PI3K gamma-deficient mice have reduced levels of allergen-induced eosinophilic inflammation and airway remodeling. Am J Physiol Lung Cell Mol Physiol 2009;296:L210–L219.
17 Pinho V, Souza DG, Barsante MM, Hamer FP, De Freitas MS, Rossi AG, Teixeira MM: Phosphoinositide-3 kinases critically regulate the recruitment and survival of eosinophils in vivo: importance for the resolution of allergic inflammation. J Leukoc Biol 2005; 77:800–810.
18 Fruman DA, Snapper SB, Yballe CM, Davidson L, Yu JY, Alt FW, Cantley LC: Impaired B cell development and proliferation in absence of phosphoinositide 3-kinase p85alpha. Science 1999;283:393–397.
19 Suzuki H, Terauchi Y, Fujiwara M, Aizawa S, Yazaki Y, Kadowaki T, Koyasu S: Xid-like immunodeficiency in mice with disruption of the p85alpha subunit of phosphoinositide 3-kinase. Science 1999;283:390–392.
20 Salogni L, Musso T, Bosisio D, Mirolo M, Jala VR, Haribabu B, Locati M, Sozzani S: Activin A induces dendritic cell migration through the polarized release of CXC chemokine ligands 12 and 14. Blood 2009;113: 5848–5856.

21 Del Prete A, Vermi W, Dander E, Otero K, Barberis L, Luini W, Bernasconi S, Sironi M, Santoro A, Garlanda C, Facchetti F, Wymann MP, Vecchi A, Hirsch E, Mantovani A, Sozzani S: Defective dendritic cell migration and activation of adaptive immunity in PI3Kgamma-deficient mice. EMBO J 2004; 23:3505–3515.
22 Ali K, Bilancio A, Thomas M, Pearce W, Gilfillan AM, Tkaczyk C, Kuehn N, Gray A, Giddings J, Peskett E, Fox R, Bruce I, Walker C, Sawyer C, Okkenhaug K, Finan P, Vanhaesebroeck B: Essential role for the p110delta phosphoinositide 3-kinase in the allergic response. Nature 2004;431:1007–1011.
23 Ali K, Camps M, Pearce WP, Ji H, Rückle T, Kuehn N, Pasquali C, Chabert C, Rommel C, Vanhaesebroeck B: Isoform-specific functions of phosphoinositide 3-kinases: p110 delta but not p110 gamma promotes optimal allergic responses in vivo. J Immunol 2008; 180:2538–2544.
24 Endo D, Gon Y, Nunomura S, Yamashita K, Hashimoto S, Ra C: PI3Kγ differentially regulates FcεRI-mediated degranulation and migration of mast cells by and toward antigen. Int Arch Allergy Immunol 2009;149: 66–72.
25 Sasaki T, Irie-Sasaki J, Jones RG, Oliveira-dos-Santos AJ, Stanford WL, Bolon B, Wakeham A, Itie A, Bouchard D, Kozieradzki I, Joza N, Mak TW, Ohashi PS, Suzuki A, Penninger JM: Function of PI3Kγ in thymocyte development, T cell activation, and neutrophil migration. Science 2000;287:1040–1046.
26 Randis TM, Puri KD, Zhou H, Diacovo TG: Role of PI3Kdelta and PI3Kgamma in inflammatory arthritis and tissue localization of neutrophils. Eur J Immunol 2008;38: 1215–1224.
27 Doukas J, Eide L, Stebbins K, Racanelli-Layton A, Dellamary L, Martin M, Dneprovskaia E, Noronha G, Soll R, Wrasidlo W, Acevedo LM, Cheresh DA: Aerosolized phosphoinositide 3-kinase gamma/delta inhibitor TG100-115 [3-[2,4-diamino-6-(3-hydroxyphenyl)pteridin-7-yl]phenol] as a therapeutic candidate for asthma and chronic obstructive pulmonary disease. J Pharmacol Exp Ther 2009;328:758–765.
28 Lai WQ, Goh HH, Bao Z, Wong WS, Melendez AJ, Leung BP: The role of sphingosine kinase in a murine model of allergic asthma. J Immunol 2008;180:4323–4329.
29 Thomas M, Edwards MJ, Sawicka E, Duggan N, Hirsch E, Wymann MP, Owen C, Trifilieff A, Walker C, Westwick J, Finan P: Essential role of phosphoinositide 3-kinase gamma in eosinophil chemotaxis within acute pulmonary inflammation. Immunology 2009;126:413–422.

Review

International Archives of Allergy and Immunology

Int Arch Allergy Immunol 2010;152(suppl 1):96–100
DOI: 10.1159/000312133

Published online: June 4, 2010

Effect of the Hepatocyte Growth Factor on Allergic Inflammatory Cells

Wataru Ito Masahide Takeda Shigeharu Ueki Tomomi Tanigai
Hiroyuki Kayaba Junichi Chihara

Department of Infection, Allergy, Clinical Immunology and Laboratory Medicine, Akita University Graduate School of Medicine, Akita, Japan

Key Words
Allergy · Asthma · Eosinophils · Hepatocyte growth factor

Abstract
Hepatocyte growth factor (HGF) has multiple activities in a variety of tissues, and is known to prevent the onset and progression of various diseases, but the mechanisms by which HGF exert its beneficial effects remain to be elucidated, although many studies have shown that HGF exerts anti-inflammatory effects in multiple animal models of diseases of the liver, kidney, lung and other organs. Recently, we have reported that HGF also reduces allergic airway inflammation in a murine model of asthma by ovalbumin. Furthermore, HGF directly modulates various functions of eosinophils, which have been shown to play a pivotal role in the development of allergic airway inflammation. HGF influences a number of cell types, and regulates various biological activities, including cytokine production, cell migration, proliferation and survival. This review focuses on the effect of HGF on various inflammatory cells, e.g. eosinophils and dendritic cells, in allergic reactions.

Allergic Diseases and Hepatocyte Growth Factor

Hepatocyte growth factor (HGF) was originally identified and cloned as a potent mitogen for mature hepatocytes [1, 2]. HGF is composed of a 69-kDa α-chain and a 34-kDa β-chain linked by a disulfide bridge. The α-chain includes an N-terminal hairpin domain and a sequence of four kringle domains, while the β-chain has a serine protease-like domain [3, 4]. HGF has many functions such as induction of angiogenesis, promotion of cell proliferation, migration and suppression of apoptosis. Therefore, HGF is now recognized as a multifunctional cytokine and/or a potent stimulator of a variety of cell types [1, 5], and there is much support that HGF plays an essential part in parenchymal repair and protection in various organs. For example, HGF prevents the onset and progression of hepatic fibrosis/cirrhosis [6], and renal [7], lung [8] and myocardial fibrosis [9] in vivo. Therefore, it was suggested that the suppressive effect of HGF on transforming growth-beta (TGF-β) plays an important role in disease progression. Furthermore, other studies have reported that HGF may be of benefit in the treatment of arteriosclerosis obliterans [10], neuronal death following cerebral ischemia [11], amyotrophic lateral sclerosis [12], gastric ulcer [13], diabetes [14], osteoarthritic

KARGER

Fax +41 61 306 12 34
E-Mail karger@karger.ch
www.karger.com

1018–2438/10/1525–0096$26.00/0

Accessible online at:
www.karger.com/iaa

Correspondence to: Dr. Junichi Chihara
Department of Infection, Allergy, Clinical Immunology and Laboratory Medicine
Akita University Graduate School of Medicine
1-1-1, Hondo, Akita 010-8543 (Japan)
Tel. +81 18 884 6180, Fax +81 18 836 2624, E-Mail chihara@hos.akita-u.ac.jp

cartilage [15] and pulmonary emphysema [16]. Recently, we and another group have reported that HGF attenuates the development of airway hyperresponsiveness, allergic airway inflammation and airway remodeling [17, 18]; in a murine model of asthma, treatment with HGF attenuated the accumulation of eosinophils and lymphocytes in peribronchial areas of the lung. Further, Th2 cytokine levels as well as growth factors such as TGF-β and platelet-derived growth factor were decreased in bronchoalveolar lavage fluid in HGF-treated mice. The HGF receptor c-Met, a product of c-Met proto-oncogene, belongs to a tyrosine kinase receptor superfamily which has been shown to regulate [19] a wide spectrum of cellular targets in multiple ways [20]. This HGF/c-Met axis plays an essential role in organ development and is pivotal in promoting tissue regeneration in injured organs [21]; c-Met protein is more prominent in acute hepatitis [22] or acute renal failure [23]. In cases of allergic inflammation, the c-Met protein was expressed in airway epithelium [24]. Thus, the up-regulation of c-Met protein expression may amplify the activity of this HGF signaling system and promote the regeneration of airway epithelium in allergic inflammation.

Dendritic Cells, T Cells, B Cells, Monocytes and HGF

Dendritic cells (DCs) are professional antigen-presenting cells, and play a central role in regulating immune responses. Previous studies have reported that DCs are crucial in the pathogenesis of asthma, and altering their functions may be of therapeutic benefit in asthma [25]. The HGF receptor c-Met is expressed on DCs, and HGF increases migration [26, 27] and adhesion [26]. In contrast, HGF does not affect DC function in the presence of antigen. Moreover, in a study by Okunishi et al. [18] in a murine model of asthma, treatment with HGF potently suppressed the ability of DCs to present antigen, thus down-regulating the supposed antigen-induced Th1- and Th2-type immune responses. Iwasaki et al. [28] also found that HGF inhibited IL-4 production in TSK (tight-skin)+ CD4+ T cells stimulated with allogeneic DCs in a murine model of scleroderma.

The c-Met transcripts are expressed in fetal and neonatal murine thymus. However, mature T cells appeared not to express c-Met. In a report by Adams et al. [29] HGF induced adhesion and migration of T cells. On the other hand, HGF inhibited T-cell proliferation as well as IL-5 production in a murine model of asthma [18], and suppressed Th2 immune responses in a murine lupus model of chronic graft-versus-host disease [30]. Moreover, Okunishi et al. reported that HGF also inhibited Th1 immune responses, e.g. IFN-γ production, in a murine model of collagen-induced arthritis [31]. Interestingly, HGF ameliorated the progression of experimental autoimmune myocarditis by inducing Th2 cytokine production from CD4+ T cells [32]. Furthermore, we found that administration of exogenous HGF to allergen-sensitized and challenged IFN-γ-deficient mice failed to affect the elevated Th2 cytokine levels in bronchoalveolar lavage fluid [17]. IFN-γ was also noted to prevent persistence of airway inflammation induced by acute allergen challenge. These findings suggest that HGF-mediated regulation of allergic airway inflammation and Th2 cytokine production may, at least in part, take place through the induction of IFN-γ production. In human B cells, HGF has been reported to influence both survival [33] and adhesion [34], while enhancing immunoglobulin production by murine lymphocytes [35]. On the other hand, substitution of stromal cells with HGF failed to enhance secretion of immunoglobulin [34]. The effects of HGF on DCs, T cells and B cells are not consistent. The divergent results seen in these studies may be related to the different cell types, experimental conditions or diseases. Mizuno et al. [36] reported HGF-induced apoptosis of myofibroblasts in lung fibrosis, whereas Zeng et al. [37] noted HGF-induced inhibition of cancer cell apoptosis. Thus, further studies are necessary to clarify the exact physiological role of HGF.

In monocytes, c-Met expression is selectively induced and functionally active. HGF induces directional migration and cytokine secretion in human monocytes [38]. On the other hand, HGF abrogates monocyte adhesion to TNF-activated endothelial monolayers [39]. Interestingly, secretion of HGF by activated monocytes is also detected, implying that monocyte function may be regulated by HGF in an autocrine as well as paracrine manner [40].

Eosinophils and HGF

Eosinophils also play a pivotal role in the development of allergic airway inflammation and airway remodeling. Human eosinophils have been shown to play very important roles in the pathogenesis of allergic inflammation by chemotaxis of inflammatory cells, production of reactive oxygen species and release of eosinophilic granule proteins. To define the direct effects of HGF on chemotactic regulation of eosinophils, we examined whether HGF has

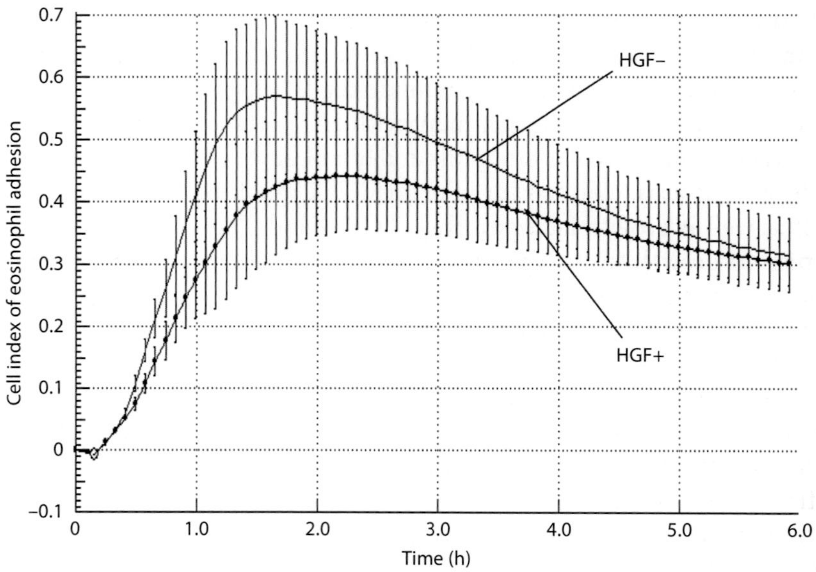

Fig. 1. HGF attenuates eosinophil adhesion. To evaluate the effects of HGF on eosinophil adhesion, a real-time assay of adhesion was performed using the xCELLigence System (Roche Applied Science), which monitors cellular events in real time by measuring electrical impedance across interdigitated micro-electrodes integrated in a culture plate coated with bovine serum albumin. To identify eosinophil adhesion by β_2-integrin to endothelial ICAM-1, BSA-coated plates were used as described [43]. This impedance measurement provides quantitative information on cell adhesion. Preincubation with 20 ng/ml HGF (HGF+) attenuated the cell index of eosinophil adhesion.

Table 1. Effects of HGF on hematopoietic cell functions

Cell	Function	Effect	Health or disease
DC	activation	↓	allergy (mouse), scleroderma (mouse)
	adhesion	↑	allergy (mouse)
	cytokine production	↓	allergy (mouse)
T cell	migration	↑	health (human)
	adhesion	↑	health (human)
	proliferation	↓	health (human), autoimmune myocarditis (mouse)
	Th1 cytokine production	↓	arthritis (mouse), lupus (mouse)
	Th1 cytokine production	↓	autoimmune myocarditis (mouse)
	Th2 cytokine production	↓	arthritis (mouse), lupus (mouse)
	Th2 cytokine production	↑	autoimmune myocarditis (mouse)
B cell	survival	↑	health (mouse)
	adhesion	↑	health (mouse)
	immunoglobulin production	↑	health (mouse)
	immunoglobulin production	→	lymphoma (human)
Monocyte	migration	↑	health (human)
	adhesion	↓	renal failure (human)
	cytokine production	↑	health (human)
Eosinophil	migration	↓	allergy (human)
	survival	→	allergy (human)
	degranulation	↓	allergy (human)
	ROS production	↓	allergy (human)
	adhesion	↓	allergy (human)

ROS = Reactive oxygen species.

any influence on eotaxin-induced migration of human purified eosinophils in the absence of cytokines such as IL-4 and IL-5. We found that HGF treatment attenuated the eotaxin-induced chemotaxis of eosinophils [41]. Further, HGF treatment suppressed the production of reactive oxygen species and eosinophil-derived neurotoxin release from activated human eosinophils [42]. Moreover, a decrease in extracellular signal-regulated kinase 1/2 and p38 mitogen-activated protein kinase signaling as well as the enhancement of Ca^{2+} influx, which are indispensable for eosinophil activation, were attenuated by HGF treatment. HGF treatment tended to inhibit adhesion of eosinophils (fig. 1). These data may indicate that HGF negatively regulated allergic airway inflammation not only through suppression of Th2 cytokine production from T cells but also via a direct action on eosinophil function, although HGF did not affect eosinophil survival in another study [41].

We have not found c-Met mRNA in either non-treated eosinophils or eosinophils stimulated with eotaxin or IL-5. Moreover, the anti-c-Met antibody failed to reverse the inhibitory effect of HGF on eosinophil migration, suggesting that c-Met is not expressed on eosinophils. Consistent with our findings, Adams et al. [29] have detected tyrosine phosphorylation in T cells in response to HGF but could not detect c-Met protein or transcripts by either PCR or Northern blotting in T cells. The mechanism by which HGF suppresses eosinophil function has only partly been elucidated. Like other growth factors, HGF binds to cell surface heparin sulfate proteoglycans that serve as low-affinity receptors and modulate HGF actions [43].

Conclusion

HGF regulates various immune cell functions including migration, adhesion, proliferation and cytokine production. Since HGF responses differ depending on the condition or cell type (table 1), HGF remains a conundrum. Although HGF has also been recognized as a homeostatic mediator that restores normal conditions in the organism, the biological potential of HGF is extremely obscure in the case of immune responses. Thus, further studies are necessary to clarify the exact mechanisms of action of HGF in allergic diseases.

Disclosure Statement

The authors declare that no financial or other conflict of interest exists in relation to the content of this article.

References

1 Nakamura T, Nawa K, Ichihara A, Kaise N, Nishino T: Purification and subunit structure of hepatocyte growth factor from rat platelets. FEBS Lett 1987;224:311–316.
2 Nakamura T, Teramoto H, Ichihara A: Purification and characterization of a growth factor from rat platelets for mature parenchymal hepatocytes in primary cultures. Proc Natl Acad Sci USA 1986;83:6489–6493.
3 Nakamura T, Nishizawa T, Hagiya M, Seki T, Shimonishi M, Sugimura A, Tashiro K, Shimizu S: Molecular cloning and expression of human hepatocyte growth factor. Nature 1989;342:440–443.
4 Miyazawa K, Tsubouchi H, Naka D, Takahashi K, Okigaki M, Arakaki N, Nakayama H, Hirono S, Sakiyama O, Takahashi K: Molecular cloning and sequence analysis of cDNA for human hepatocyte growth factor. Biochem Biophys Res Commun 1989;163:967–973.
5 Matsumoto K, Nakamura T: Emerging multipotent aspects of hepatocyte growth factor. J Biochem 1996;119:591–600.
6 Ueki T, Kaneda Y, Tsutsui H, Nakanishi K, Sawa Y, Morishita R, Matsumoto K, Nakamura T, Takahashi H, Okamoto E, Fujimoto J: Hepatocyte growth factor gene therapy of liver cirrhosis in rats. Nat Med 1999;5:226–230.
7 Mizuno S, Kurosawa T, Matsumoto K, Mizuno-Horikawa Y, Okamoto M, Nakamura T: Hepatocyte growth factor prevents renal fibrosis and dysfunction in a mouse model of chronic renal disease. J Clin Invest 1998;101:1827–1834.
8 Taniyama Y, Morishita R, Nakagami H, Moriguchi A, Sakonjo H, Shokei-Kim, Matsumoto K, Nakamura T, Higaki J, Ogihara T: Potential contribution of a novel antifibrotic factor, hepatocyte growth factor, to prevention of myocardial fibrosis by angiotensin II blockade in cardiomyopathic hamsters. Circulation 2000;102:246–252.
9 Yaekashiwa M, Nakayama S, Ohnuma K, Sakai T, Abe T, Satoh K, Matsumoto K, Nakamura T, Takahashi T, Nukiwa T: Simultaneous or delayed administration of hepatocyte growth factor equally represses the fibrotic changes in murine lung injury induced by bleomycin. A morphologic study. Am J Respir Crit Care Med 1997;156:1937–1944.
10 Taniyama Y, Morishita R, Hiraoka K, Aoki M, Nakagami H, Yamasaki K, Matsumoto K, Nakamura T, Kaneda Y, Ogihara T: Therapeutic angiogenesis induced by human hepatocyte growth factor gene in rat diabetic hind limb ischemia model: molecular mechanisms of delayed angiogenesis in diabetes. Circulation 2001;104:2344–2350.
11 Miyazawa T, Matsumoto K, Ohmichi H, Katoh H, Yamashima T, Nakamura T: Protection of hippocampal neurons from ischemia-induced delayed neuronal death by hepatocyte growth factor: a novel neurotrophic factor. J Cereb Blood Flow Metab 1998;18:345–348.

12 Sun W, Funakoshi H, Nakamura T: Overexpression of HGF retards disease progression and prolongs life span in a transgenic mouse model of ALS. J Neurosci 2002;22:6537–6548.
13 Brzozowski T, Konturek PC, Konturek SJ, Schuppan D, Drozdowicz D, Kwiecien S, Majka J, Nakamura T, Hahn E: Effect of local application of growth factors on gastric ulcer healing and mucosal expression of cyclooxygenase-1 and -2. Digestion 2001;64:15–29.
14 Dai C, Li Y, Yang J, Liu Y: Hepatocyte growth factor preserves beta cell mass and mitigates hyperglycemia in streptozotocin-induced diabetic mice. J Biol Chem 2003;278:27080–27087.
15 Reboul P, Pelletier JP, Tardif G, Benderdour M, Ranger P, Bottaro DP, Martel-Pelletier J: Hepatocyte growth factor induction of collagenase 3 production in human osteoarthritic cartilage: involvement of the stress-activated protein kinase/c-Jun N-terminal kinase pathway and a sensitive p38 mitogen-activated protein kinase inhibitor cascade. Arthritis Rheum 2001;44:73–84.
16 Shigemura N, Sawa Y, Mizuno S, Ono M, Ohta M, Nakamura T, Kaneda Y, Matsuda H: Amelioration of pulmonary emphysema by in vivo gene transfection with hepatocyte growth factor in rats. Circulation 2005;111:1407–1414.
17 Ito W, Kanehiro A, Matsumoto K, Hirano A, Ono K, Maruyama H, Kataoka M, Nakamura T, Gelfand EW, Tanimoto M: Hepatocyte growth factor attenuates airway hyperresponsiveness, inflammation, and remodeling. Am J Respir Cell Mol Biol 2005;32:268–280.
18 Okunishi K, Dohi M, Nakagome K, Tanaka R, Mizuno S, Matsumoto K, Miyazaki J, Nakamura T, Yamamoto K: A novel role of hepatocyte growth factor as an immune regulator through suppressing dendritic cell function. J Immunol 2005;175:4745–4753.
19 Bottaro DP, Rubin JS, Faletto DL, Chan AM, Kmiecik TE, Vande Woude GF, Aaronson SA: Identification of the hepatocyte growth factor receptor as the c-met proto-oncogene product. Science 1991;251:802–804.
20 Rubin JS, Bottaro DP, Aaronson SA: Hepatocyte growth factor/scatter factor and its receptor, the c-met proto-oncogene product. Biochim Biophys Acta 1993;1155:357–371.
21 Ishiki Y, Ohnishi H, Muto Y, Matsumoto K, Nakamura T: Direct evidence that hepatocyte growth factor is a hepatotrophic factor for liver regeneration and has a potent antihepatitis effect in vivo. Hepatology 1992;16:1227–1235.
22 Okano J, Shiota G, Kawasaki H: Expression of hepatocyte growth factor (HGF) and HGF receptor (c-met) proteins in liver diseases: an immunohistochemical study. Liver 1999;19:151–159.
23 Liu Y, Tolbert EM, Lin L, Thursby MA, Sun AM, Nakamura T, Dworkin LD: Up-regulation of hepatocyte growth factor receptor: an amplification and targeting mechanism for hepatocyte growth factor action in acute renal failure. Kidney Int 1999;55:442–453.
24 Ito W, Tanimoto M, Ono K, Mizuno S, Yoshida A, Koga H, Fuchimoto Y, Kondo N, Tanimoto Y, Kiura K, Matsumoto K, Kataoka M, Nakamura T, Gelfand EW, Kanehiro A: Growth factors temporally associate with airway responsiveness and inflammation in allergen-exposed mice. Int Arch Allergy Immunol 2008;145:324–339.
25 Lambrecht BN, Hammad H: Taking our breath away: dendritic cells in the pathogenesis of asthma. Nat Rev Immunol 2003;3:994–1003.
26 Kurz SM, Diebold SS, Hieronymus T, Gust TC, Bartunek P, Sachs M, Birchmeier W, Zenke M: The impact of c-met/scatter factor receptor on dendritic cell migration. Eur J Immunol 2002;32:1832–1838.
27 Scarpino S, Stoppacciaro A, Ballerini F, Marchesi M, Prat M, Stella MC, Sozzani S, Allavena P, Mantovani A, Ruco LP: Papillary carcinoma of the thyroid: hepatocyte growth factor (HGF) stimulates tumor cells to release chemokines active in recruiting dendritic cells. Am J Pathol 2000;156:831–837.
28 Iwasaki T, Imado T, Kitano S, Sano H: Hepatocyte growth factor ameliorates dermal sclerosis in the tight-skin mouse model of scleroderma. Arthritis Res Ther 2006;8:R161.
29 Adams DH, Harvath L, Bottaro DP, Interrante R, Catalano G, Tanaka Y, Strain A, Hubscher SG, Shaw S: Hepatocyte growth factor and macrophage inflammatory protein 1 beta: structurally distinct cytokines that induce rapid cytoskeletal changes and subset-preferential migration in T cells. Proc Natl Acad Sci USA 1994;91:7144–7148.
30 Kuroiwa T, Iwasaki T, Imado T, Sekiguchi M, Fujimoto J, Sano H: Hepatocyte growth factor prevents lupus nephritis in a murine lupus model of chronic graft-versus-host disease. Arthritis Res Ther 2006;8:R123.
31 Okunishi K, Dohi M, Fujio K, Nakagome K, Tabata Y, Okasora T, Seki M, Shibuya M, Imamura M, Harada H, Tanaka R, Yamamoto K: Hepatocyte growth factor significantly suppresses collagen-induced arthritis in mice. J Immunol 2007;179:5504–5513.
32 Futamatsu H, Suzuki J, Mizuno S, Koga N, Adachi S, Kosuge H, Maejima Y, Hirao K, Nakamura T, Isobe M: Hepatocyte growth factor ameliorates the progression of experimental autoimmune myocarditis: a potential role for induction of T helper 2 cytokines. Circ Res 2005;96:823–830.
33 Skibinski G, Skibinska A, James K: The role of hepatocyte growth factor and its receptor c-met in interactions between lymphocytes and stromal cells in secondary human lymphoid organs. Immunology 2001;102:506–514.
34 van der Voort R, Taher TE, Keehnen RM, Smit L, Groenink M, Pals ST: Paracrine regulation of germinal center B cell adhesion through the c-met-hepatocyte growth factor/scatter factor pathway. J Exp Med 1997;185:2121–2131.
35 Delaney B, Koh WS, Yang KH, Strom SC, Kaminski NE: Hepatocyte growth factor enhances B-cell activity. Life Sci 1993;53:PL89–PL93.
36 Mizuno S, Matsumoto K, Li MY, Nakamura T: HGF reduces advancing lung fibrosis in mice: a potential role for MMP-dependent myofibroblast apoptosis. FASEB J 2005;19:580–582.
37 Zeng Q, Chen S, You Z, Yang F, Carey TE, Saims D, Wang CY: Hepatocyte growth factor inhibits anoikis in head and neck squamous cell carcinoma cells by activation of ERK and Akt signaling independent of NF kappa B. J Biol Chem 2002;277:25203–25208.
38 Galimi F, Cottone E, Vigna E, Arena N, Boccaccio C, Giordano S, Naldini L, Comoglio PM: Hepatocyte growth factor is a regulator of monocyte-macrophage function. J Immunol 2001;166:1241–1247.
39 Gong R, Rifai A, Dworkin LD: Anti-inflammatory effect of hepatocyte growth factor in chronic kidney disease: targeting the inflamed vascular endothelium. J Am Soc Nephrol 2006;17:2464–2473.
40 Skibinski G: The role of hepatocyte growth factor/c-met interactions in the immune system. Arch Immunol Ther Exp (Warsz) 2003;51:277–282.
41 Ito W, Chiba T, Kanehiro A, Kato H, Yamaguchi K, Ueki S, Kayaba H, Chihara J: Hepatocyte growth factor attenuates eotaxin and PGD2-induced chemotaxis of human eosinophils. Allergy 2007;62:415–422.
42 Ito W, Takeda M, Fujita M, Kamada Y, Kato H, Chiba T, Yamaguchi K, Ueki S, Kayaba H, Kanehiro A, Chihara J: Hepatocyte growth factor suppresses production of reactive oxygen species and release of eosinophil-derived neurotoxin from human eosinophils. Int Arch Allergy Immunol 2008;147:331–337.
43 Rubin JS, Day RM, Breckenridge D, Atabey N, Taylor WG, Stahl SJ, Wingfield PT, Kaufman JD, Schwall R, Bottaro DP: Dissociation of heparan sulfate and receptor binding domains of hepatocyte growth factor reveals that heparan sulfate-c-met interaction facilitates signaling. J Biol Chem 2001;276:32977–32983.

Review

International Archives of Allergy and Immunology

Int Arch Allergy Immunol 2010;152(suppl 1):101–105
DOI: 10.1159/000312134

Published online: June 4, 2010

FIP1L1/PDGFRα-Associated Systemic Mastocytosis

Yoshiyuki Yamada[a] Jose A. Cancelas[b]

[a]Division of Allergy and Immunology, Gunma Children's Medical Center, Shibukawa, Gunma, Japan;
[b]Division of Experimental Hematology, Department of Pediatrics, Cincinnati Children's Hospital Medical Center, and Hoxworth Blood Center, University of Cincinnati College of Medicine, Cincinnati, Ohio, USA

Key Words
Chronic eosinophilic leukemia · Eosinophils · FIP1L1/PDGFRα · Hypereosinophilic syndromes · Interleukin-5 · Mast cells · Stem cell factor · Systemic mastocytosis

Abstract
Since the identification of the *FIP1L1/PDGFRA* fusion gene as a pathogenic cause of the hypereosinophilic syndrome (HES), the importance of the molecular classification of HES leading to the diagnosis of chronic eosinophilic leukemia (CEL) has been recognized. As a result, a new category, 'myeloid and lymphoid neoplasm with eosinophilia and abnormalities in PDGFRA, PDGFRB or FGFR1', has recently been added to the new WHO criteria for myeloid neoplasms. FIP1L1/PDGFRα-positive disorders are characterized by clonal hypereosinophilia, multiple organ dysfunctions due to eosinophil infiltration, systemic mastocytosis (SM) and a dramatic response to treatment with imatinib mesylate. A murine HES/CEL model by the introduction of FIP1L1/PDGFRα and IL-5 overexpression also shows SM, representing patients with FIP1L1/PDGFRα-positive HES/CEL/SM. The murine model and the in vitro development system of FIP1L1/PDGFRα-positive mast cells revealed the interaction between FIP1L1/PDGFRα, IL-5 and stem cell factor in the development of HES/CEL/SM. Current findings of FIP1L1/PDGFRα-positive HES/CEL are reviewed focusing on aberrant mast cell development leading to SM.

Introduction

The importance of the molecular classification of the hypereosinophilic syndrome (HES) has been increasingly recognized. The fusion gene *FIP1L1/PDGFRA* was identified in a large number of patients initially diagnosed as having a myeloproliferative variant of HES or chronic eosinophilic leukemia (CEL) [1]. Subsequently, other variant PDGFRA fusion genes as well as those involving PDGFRB or FGFR1 have also been described in myeloproliferative neoplasms with eosinophilia in the last years [2–4]. As a result, a new category of myeloid neoplasms, 'myeloid and lymphoid neoplasm with eosinophilia and abnormalities of PDGFRA, PDGFRB or FGFR1', has recently been added to the new WHO criteria [5]. FIP1L1/PDGFRα fusion-positive disorders are characterized by clonal myeloproliferation resulting in hypereosinophilia, multiple organ dysfunctions due to eosinophil infiltration, a dramatic response to treatment with

KARGER

Fax +41 61 306 12 34
E-Mail karger@karger.ch
www.karger.com

Accessible online at:
www.karger.com/iaa

Correspondence to: Dr. Yoshiyuki Yamada
Division of Allergy and Immunology
Gunma Children's Medical Center
779 Shimohakoda, Hokkitsu, Shibukawa, Gunma 377-8577 (Japan)
Tel. +81 279 52 3551, Fax +81 279 52 2045, E-Mail yamaday@gcmc.pref.gunma.jp

imatinib mesylate and systemic mastocytosis (SM) [6]. Murine models of FIP1L1/PDGFRα-induced diseases have been reported recently [7, 8]. Interestingly, these models demonstrated severe SM representing patients with FIP1L1/PDGFRα fusion-positive diseases [9]. In this review, the clinical manifestation of FIP1L1/PDGFRα fusion-associated disorders are summarized, focusing on mastocytosis induced by FIP1L1/PDGFRα expression, and the mechanisms of mastocytosis in FIP1L1/PDGFRα-positive HES/CEL are discussed.

Eosinophilia in SM Patients

Peripheral blood eosinophilia has been reported in 15–28% of SM patients [10–12]. This is no big surprise since crosstalk between eosinophils and mast cells is well known, especially in allergic inflammation. For instance, mast cell activation by major basic protein, an eosinophil granule protein, elicits the generation of lipid mediators and cytokines. Eosinophils also produce cytokines associated with mast cell activation such as stem cell factor (SCF), granulocyte/macrophage colony-stimulating factor and nerve growth factor [13]. The D816V mutation in the *KIT* gene resulting in constitutive activation of the receptor tyrosine kinase has been shown in the majority of patients as a cause of SM [14]. D816V-kit mutation-positive SM with eosinophilia has been clinically distinguished from that without eosinophilia. D816V-kit mutation-positive SM patients with eosinophilia present hepatosplenomegaly, lymphadenopathy, anemia and monocytosis more frequently as well as higher levels of circulating tryptase, whereas anaphylaxis is seen with a low frequency in these patients, in comparison to patients without eosinophilia [10].

Clinical Manifestations of Mastocytosis Associated with FIP1L1/PDGFRα

A recent report has shown that FIP1L1/PDGFRα-associated SM is a clinically distinguishable disease from D816V mutation SM with eosinophilia [10]. FIP1L1/PDGFRα-associated SM shows lower tryptase levels in the circulation, less aggregation of bone marrow mast cells, more severe eosinophilia, higher serum vitamin B12 levels and more frequent pulmonary and cardiac involvement than D816V SM with associated eosinophilia. The clinical difference is important since it would justify the differential diagnosis between these two entities, based on the analysis of the expression of the FIP1L1/*PDGFRA* fusion gene. More recently, Klion [15] proposed a scoring system to approach FIP1L1/PDGFRα fusion-positive HES/CEL therapy appropriately.

SM in Murine Models of FIP1L1/PDGFRα-Positive Disorders

First, Cools et al. [7] reported that the introduction of the *FIP1L1/PDGFRA* fusion gene into bone marrow hematopoietic stem cells and progenitors (HSC/P) induces a murine model of a myeloproliferative disorder (MPD) similar to that found in p210-BCR/ABL-induced chronic myelogenous leukemia-like disease (F/P-MPD). Subsequently, an HES/CEL murine model was developed by the introduction of the *FIP1L1/PDGFRA* fusion gene into bone marrow HSC/Ps in the presence of T-cell overexpression of IL-5 (F/P-HES/CEL) [8]. More recently, these two murine models were also shown to develop tissue mast cell infiltration and increased circulating mast cell protease 1 (MMCP-1) levels, which is a systemic assay of mast cell content and degranulation in the mouse resembling serum tryptase determination in SM patients [9]. Similar to the patients with *FIP1L1/PDGFRA* fusion gene, tissue mast cell infiltration of hematopoietic organs, skin and intestine, where mast cell morphology is aberrant, is present in F/P-HES/CEL mice. Tissue mast cell shape is irregular with frequent cytoplasmic extensions reminiscent of the 'spindle shape' found in clinical SM. In addition, serum levels of MMCP-1 are extremely elevated in F/P-HES/CEL mice.

A possible interaction of IL-5 with the SM phenotype was analyzed in F/P-HES/CEL mice. F/P-HES/CEL and F/P-MPD mice showed significantly greater mast cell infiltration in their skin and intestine, and higher levels of MMCP-1 compared to both controls with and without IL-5 overexpression. Interestingly, intestinal mast cell infiltration and serum MMCP-1 levels in F/P-HES/CEL mice were significantly higher compared to F/P-MPD, suggesting that FIP1L1/PDGFRα in conjunction with IL-5 exacerbates mastocytosis in murine F/P-HES/CEL [9].

Mechanism of FIP1L1/PDGFRα-Promoted Mast Cell Development

Since the c-kit signaling pathway is pivotal for normal mast cell development and function, the question of whether FIP1L1/PDGFRα-associated SM is still c-kit de-

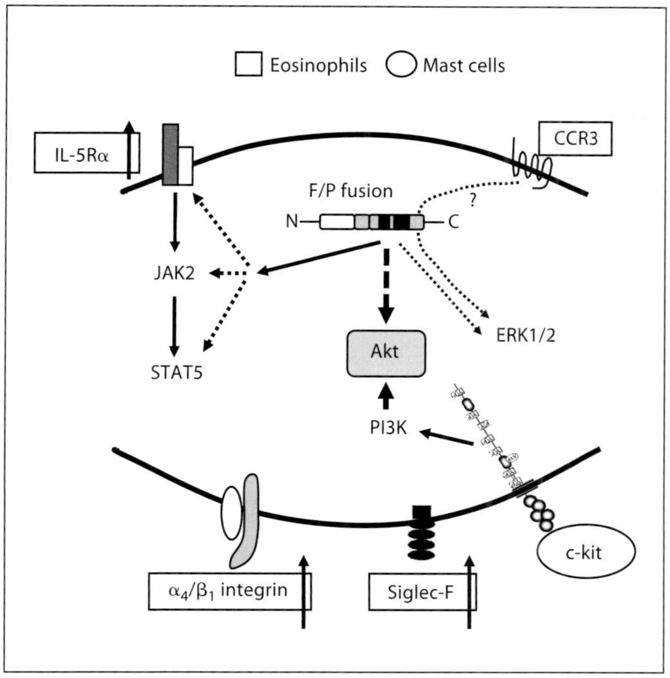

Fig. 1. Intracellular signaling of FIP1L1/PDGFRα+ (F/P) cells. FIP1L1/PDGFRα+ (F/P) primary mouse eosinophils express up-regulated IL-5Rα and FIP1L1/PDGFRα activates the JAK2/STAT5 pathway. The CCR3/ERK1/2 signaling pathway may be amplified by FIP1L1/PDGFRα expression [25]. Up-regulated expressions of α_4 integrin and Siglec-F were observed in FIP1L1/PDGFRα+ murine eosinophils [8]. FIP1L1/PDGFRα synergizes with SCF stimulation via c-kit to activate Akt signaling in mouse mast cells. Eosinophils and mast cells also express c-kit and IL-5Rα, respectively.

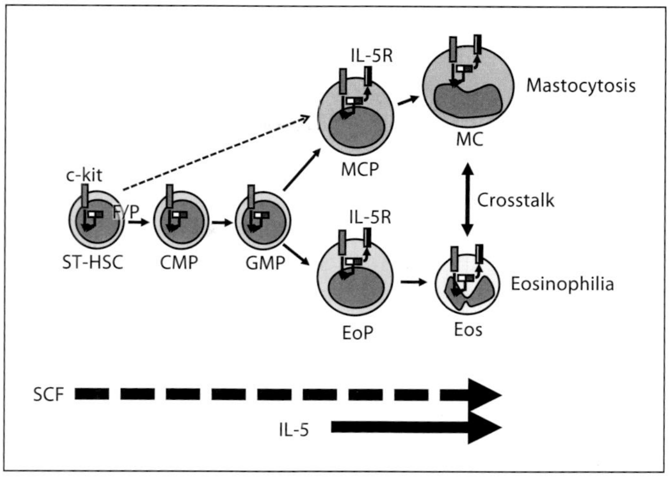

Fig. 2. FIP1L1/PDGFRα in conjunction with SCF and IL-5 promote leukemic hematopoiesis and eosinophil and mast cell (MC) development. FIP1L1/PDGFRα may occur in hematopoietic stem cells or early progenitor cells resulting in the expression of FIP1L1/PDGFRα in most hematopoietic cells. Progenitors including earlier and mature eosinophils and MCs express c-kit. In contrast, IL-5Rα expression has been observed on eosinophil progenitor (EoP), MC progenitor (MCP) and mature eosinophils and MCs. FIP1L1/PDGFRα enhances SCF/c-kit signaling by sharing downstream signaling and up-regulates IL-5Rα expression facilitating its intracellular signaling. There is significant crosstalk between eosinophils and MCs. These findings imply that FIP1L1/PDGFRα in collaboration with SCF may affect leukemic myeloproliferation, and synergistically with IL-5 expand and activate MC and eosinophil lineages. ST-HSC = Short-term HSC; CMP = common myeloid progenitor; GMP = granulocyte-macrophage progenitor.

pendent arises. In fact, following blockade of the the c-kit signaling pathway using anti-c-kit antibody, tissue mast cells and circulating levels of MMCP-1 were significantly decreased, suggesting that tissue infiltration of FIP1L1/PDGFRα fusion-positive mast cells are associated with SCF/c-kit signaling. The ex vivo cytokine-dependent mast cell differentiation of FIP1L1/PDGFRα-expressing HSC/Ps was largely dependent on the use of SCF in the culture conditions. Moreover, FIP1L1/PDGFRα fusion-positive mast cells showed prolonged survival and enhanced migration toward SCF. Specific synergistic stimulation of the Akt signaling pathway by FIP1L1/PDGFRα and SCF indicated collaboration of two tyrosine kinase activities in their downstream signaling pathways. Taken together, FIP1L1/PDGFRα synergizes with the SCF/c-kit pathway to promote mast cell development, activation and survival both in vivo and in vitro [9].

Pathogenesis of FIP1L1/PDGFRα-Positive HES/CEL/SM Associated with SCF and IL-5

Previously, we reported that the induction of murine HES/CEL by FIP1L1/PDGFRα requires a second event that is associated with IL-5 overexpression [8]. In addition, the level of expression of IL-5Rα was exclusively up-regulated in FIP1L1/PDGFRα-positive splenocytes and FIP1L1/PDGFRα fusion protein shares the downstream JAK2/STAT5 pathway with IL-5 signaling (fig. 1) [16]. Interestingly, polymorphisms of the human *IL-5RA* gene have been found linked to the constitutional *IL-5RA* genotype and the severity of FIP1L1/PDGFRα-positive CEL [17]. These findings suggest that amplification of IL-5 signaling by FIP1L1/PDGFRα triggers a CEL-like disease. Interestingly, IL-5Rα is expressed on eosinophil and mast cell progenitors [18, 19] as well as mature eosinophils [20] and mast cells [21], whereas c-kit expression is not only found on progenitors but also on mature eosinophils and mast cells [14, 18, 19]. Importantly, expression of the *FIP1L1/PDGFRA* fusion gene or deletion of the surrogate marker CHIC2 have been detected in non-eosinophilic cells, including neutrophils, monocytes, mast cells, lymphoid lineage cells and bone marrow CD34-positive cells in part of the patients, suggesting that the fusion of the *FIP1L1/PDGFRA* genes may occur in HSCs or early progenitors [22–24]. Taken together, these findings imply that FIP1L1/PDGFRα in collaboration with SCF may affect leukemic myeloproliferation and synergistically with IL-5 expand and activate mast cell and eosinophil lineages (fig. 2).

Conclusion

HES/CEL has attracted a lot of attention since the patients were successfully treated with imatinib mesylate, and subsequently the target, FIP1L1/PDGFRα, was discovered in a large number of patients initially diagnosed as myeloproliferative variant of HES. To our knowledge, there is little doubt that FIP1L1/PDGFRα preferentially affects eosinophil and mast cell proliferation, survival, differentiation and tissue infiltration, and leukemogenesis is induced combined with systemic or local extrinsic factors, as demonstrated by crucial roles of IL-5 and SCF in the pathogenesis of FIP1L1/PDGFRα-initiated HES/CEL/SM. This disease, an example of the crosstalk between oncogenesis and inflammation, represents an excellent model to study cellular integration of biochemical signals in cancer, being responsible for crucial aspects of cancer biology, e.g. cell proliferation, survival, tissue invasion and communication with the specific tissue microenvironment.

Acknowledgments

We are grateful to Drs. Marc E. Rothenberg (Cincinnati Children's Hospital Medical Center) and David A. Williams (Children's Hospital, Boston, Mass., USA) for their help in the development of the murine CEL/HES model. J.A.C. was supported by the National Institutes of Health (HL080759 and HL080759-01A2S1) and U.S. DoD (CM064050).

Disclosure Statement

The authors declare that no financial or other conflict of interest exists in relation to the content of this article.

References

1 Cools J, DeAngelo DJ, Gotlib J, Stover EH, Legare RD, Cortes J, Kutok J, Clark J, Galinsky I, Griffin JD, Cross NC, Tefferi A, Malone J, Alam R, Schrier SL, Schmid J, Rose M, Vandenberghe P, Verhoef G, Boogaerts M, Wlodarska I, Kantarjian H, Marynen P, Coutre SE, Stone R, Gilliland DG: A tyrosine kinase created by fusion of the PDGFRA and FIP1L1 genes as a therapeutic target of imatinib in idiopathic hypereosinophilic syndrome. N Engl J Med 2003;348:1201–1214.
2 Curtis CE, Grand FH, Musto P, Clark A, Murphy J, Perla G, Minervini MM, Stewart J, Reiter A, Cross NC: Two novel imatinib-responsive PDGFRA fusion genes in chronic eosinophilic leukaemia. Br J Haematol 2007; 138:77–81.
3 Score J, Curtis C, Waghorn K, Stalder M, Jotterand M, Grand FH, Cross NC: Identification of a novel imatinib-responsive KIF5B-PDGFRA fusion gene following screening for PDGFRA overexpression in patients with hypereosinophilia. Leukemia 2006;20:827–832.
4 Walz C, Curtis C, Schnittger S, Schultheis B, Metzgeroth G, Schoch C, Lengfelder E, Erben P, Muller MC, Haferlach T, Hochhaus A, Hehlmann R, Cross NC, Reiter A: Transient response to imatinib in a chronic eosinophilic leukemia associated with ins(9;4)(q33;q12q25) and a CDK5RAP2-PDGFRA fusion gene. Genes Chromosomes Cancer 2006;45:950–956.
5 Tefferi A, Vardiman JW: Classification and diagnosis of myeloproliferative neoplasms: the 2008 World Health Organization criteria and point-of-care diagnostic algorithms. Leukemia 2008;22:14–22.
6 Gotlib J, Cools J: Five years since the discovery of FIP1L1-PDGFRA: what we have learned about the fusion and other molecularly defined eosinophilias. Leukemia 2008; 22:1999–2010.
7 Cools J, Stover EH, Boulton CL, Gotlib J, Legare RD, Amaral SM, Curley DP, Duclos N, Rowan R, Kutok JL, Lee BH, Williams IR, Coutre SE, Stone RM, DeAngelo DJ, Marynen P, Manley PW, Meyer T, Fabbro D, Neuberg D, Weisberg E, Griffin JD, Gilliland DG: PKC412 overcomes resistance to imatinib in a murine model of FIP1L1-PDGFRalpha-induced myeloproliferative disease. Cancer Cell 2003;3:459–469.
8 Yamada Y, Rothenberg ME, Lee AW, Akei HS, Brandt EB, Williams DA, Cancelas JA: The FIP1L1-PDGFRA fusion gene cooperates with IL-5 to induce murine hypereosinophilic syndrome (HES)/chronic eosinophilic leukemia (CEL)-like disease. Blood 2006;107:4071–4079.
9 Yamada Y, Sanchez-Aguilera A, Brandt EB, McBride M, Al-Moamen NJ, Finkelman FD, Williams DA, Cancelas JA, Rothenberg ME: FIP1L1/PDGFRalpha synergizes with SCF to induce systemic mastocytosis in a murine model of chronic eosinophilic leukemia/hypereosinophilic syndrome. Blood 2008;112: 2500–2507.

10 Maric I, Robyn J, Metcalfe DD, Fay MP, Carter M, Wilson T, Fu W, Stoddard J, Scott L, Hartsell M, Kirshenbaum A, Akin C, Nutman TB, Noel P, Klion AD: KIT D816V-associated systemic mastocytosis with eosinophilia and FIP1L1/PDGFRA-associated chronic eosinophilic leukemia are distinct entities. J Allergy Clin Immunol 2007;120: 680–687.
11 Pardanani A, Reeder T, Li CY, Tefferi A: Eosinophils are derived from the neoplastic clone in patients with systemic mastocytosis and eosinophilia. Leuk Res 2003;27:883–885.
12 Lawrence JB, Friedman BS, Travis WD, Chinchilli VM, Metcalfe DD, Gralnick HR: Hematologic manifestations of systemic mast cell disease: a prospective study of laboratory and morphologic features and their relation to prognosis. Am J Med 1991;91: 612–624.
13 Rothenberg ME, Hogan SP: The eosinophil. Annu Rev Immunol 2006;24:147–174.
14 Patnaik MM, Rindos M, Kouides PA, Tefferi A, Pardanani A: Systemic mastocytosis: a concise clinical and laboratory review. Arch Pathol Lab Med 2007;131:784–791.
15 Klion AD: How I treat hypereosinophilic syndromes. Blood 2009;114:3736–3741.
16 Cools J, Quentmeier H, Huntly BJ, Marynen P, Griffin JD, Drexler HG, Gilliland DG: The EOL-1 cell line as an in vitro model for the study of FIP1L1-PDGFRA-positive chronic eosinophilic leukemia. Blood 2004;103: 2802–2805.
17 Burgstaller S, Kreil S, Waghorn K, Metzgeroth G, Preudhomme C, Zoi K, White H, Cilloni D, Zoi C, Brito-Babapulle F, Walz C, Reiter A, Cross NC: The severity of FIP1L1-PDGFRA-positive chronic eosinophilic leukaemia is associated with polymorphic variation at the IL5RA locus. Leukemia 2007;21:2428–2432.
18 Iwasaki H, Mizuno S, Mayfield R, Shigematsu H, Arinobu Y, Seed B, Gurish MF, Takatsu K, Akashi K: Identification of eosinophil lineage-committed progenitors in the murine bone marrow. J Exp Med 2005;201:1891–1897.
19 Arinobu Y, Iwasaki H, Akashi K: Origin of basophils and mast cells. Allergol Int 2009; 58:21–28.
20 Yuan Q, Austen KF, Friend DS, Heidtman M, Boyce JA: Human peripheral blood eosinophils express a functional c-kit receptor for stem cell factor that stimulates very late antigen 4 (VLA-4)-mediated cell adhesion to fibronectin and vascular cell adhesion molecule 1 (VCAM-1). J Exp Med 1997;186:313–323.
21 Dahl C, Hoffmann HJ, Saito H, Schiotz PO: Human mast cells express receptors for IL-3, IL-5 and GM-CSF; a partial map of receptors on human mast cells cultured in vitro. Allergy 2004;59:1087–1096.
22 Pardanani A, Ketterling RP, Brockman SR, Flynn HC, Paternoster SF, Shearer BM, Reeder TL, Li CY, Cross NC, Cools J, Gilliland DG, Dewald GW, Tefferi A: CHIC2 deletion, a surrogate for FIP1L1-PDGFRA fusion, occurs in systemic mastocytosis associated with eosinophilia and predicts response to imatinib mesylate therapy. Blood 2003;102:3093–3096.
23 Robyn J, Lemery S, McCoy JP, Kubofcik J, Kim YJ, Pack S, Nutman TB, Dunbar C, Klion AD: Multilineage involvement of the fusion gene in patients with FIP1L1/PDGFRA-positive hypereosinophilic syndrome. Br J Haematol 2006;132:286–292.
24 Tefferi A, Lasho TL, Brockman SR, Elliott MA, Dispenzieri A, Pardanani A: FIP1L1-PDGFRA and c-kit D816V mutation-based clonality studies in systemic mast cell disease associated with eosinophilia. Haematologica 2004;89:871–873.
25 Adachi T, Hanaka S, Yano T, Yamamura K, Yoshihara H, Nagase H, Chihara J, Ohta K: The role of platelet-derived growth factor receptor in eotaxin signaling of eosinophils. Int Arch Allergy Immunol 2006;140(suppl 1):28–34.

International Archives of
Allergy and Immunology

Int Arch Allergy Immunol 2010;152(suppl 1):106
DOI: 10.1159/000312135

Published online: June 4, 2010

List of Lectures by Speakers Who Have Not Submitted Their Manuscripts

Analysis of IL-33-Induced Allergic Airway Inflammation

Maho Suzukawa et al.

Department of Internal Medicine, Teikyo University School of Medicine, Tokyo, Japan

Examination of Useful Antitussives against Cough of *Mycoplasma pneumoniae* Bronchitis-Cough of *Mycoplasma pneumoniae* Infection May Be Considered in Eosinophilic Inflammation

Naoto Watanabe et al.

Faculty of Pharmaceutical Sciences, Laboratory of Pharmacology, Josai International University, Togane, Japan

Neuropeptides Modulate TGF-β Inducible Early Gene Expression in Both Cultured Airway Epithelial Cells and Smooth Muscle Cells

Makoto Fueki et al.

Department of Pulmonary Medicine and Clinical Immunology, Dokkyo Medical University School of Medicine, Mibu, Japan

Sex Difference in Transcriptional Regulation of Th2 Cytokine Expression in a Murine Model of Allergic Asthma

Kana Wada et al.

Department of Pathophysiology, Tohoku Pharmaceutical University, Sendai, Japan

The Roles of Fungal Antigens and *Staphylococcus aureus* Enterotoxins in Chronic Rhinosinusitis (CRS)

Yoshinori Matsuwaki et al.

Department of Otorhinolaryngology, Jikey University School of Medicine, Tokyo, Japan

KARGER

Fax +41 61 306 12 34
E-Mail karger@karger.ch
www.karger.com

1018–2438/10/1525–0106$26.00/0

Accessible online at:
www.karger.com/iaa

Author Index Vol. 152, Suppl. 1, 2010

International Archives of Allergy and Immunology

KARGER

Fax +41 61 306 12 34
E-Mail karger@karger.ch
www.karger.com

Accessible online at:
www.karger.com/iaa

Subject Index Vol. 152, Suppl. 1, 2010

International Archives of
Allergy and Immunology

KARGER
Fax +41 61 306 12 34
E-Mail karger@karger.ch
www.karger.com

Accessible online at:
www.karger.com/iaa